A Social History
of the Minor Tranquilizers

The Quest for Small Comfort in the Age of Anxiety

PHARMACEUTICAL PRODUCTS PRESS
Pharmaceutical Sciences
Mickey C. Smith, PhD
Executive Editor

New, Recent, and Forthcoming Titles:

Principles of Pharmaceutical Marketing edited by Mickey C. Smith

Pharmacy Ethics edited by Mickey C. Smith, Steven Strauss, John Baldwin, and Kelly T. Alberts

Drug-Related Problems in Geriatric Nursing Home Patients by James W. Cooper

Pharmacy and the U.S. Health Care System edited by Jack E. Fincham and Albert I. Wertheimer

Pharmaceutical Marketing: Strategy and Cases by Mickey C. Smith

International Pharmaceutical Services: The Drug Industry and Pharmacy Practice in Twenty Major Countries of the World edited by Richard N. Spivey, Albert I. Wertheimer, and T. Donald Rucker

A Social History of the Minor Tranquilizers: The Quest for Small Comfort in the Age of Anxiety by Mickey C. Smith

Marketing Pharmaceutical Services: Patron Loyalty, Satisfaction, and Preferences edited by Harry A. Smith and Stephen Joel Coons

A Social History of the Minor Tranquilizers

The Quest for Small Comfort in the Age of Anxiety

Mickey C. Smith

Pharmaceutical Products Press
An Imprint of The Haworth Press, Inc.
New York • London • Sydney

Originally published as *Small Comfort: A History of the Minor Tranquilizers*. © 1985 by Praeger Publishers.

Pharmaceutical Products Press, 10 Alice Street, Binghamton, NY 13904-1580
EUROSPAN/Pharmaceutical Products Press, 3 Henrietta Street, London WC2E 8LU England
ASTAM/Pharmaceutical Products Press, 162-168 Parramatta Road, Stanmore (Sydney), N.S.W. 2048 Australia

Pharmaceutical Products Press is an imprint of The Haworth Press, Inc., 10 Alice Street, Binghamton, NY 13904-1580.

Library of Congress Cataloging-in-Publication Data

Smith, Mickey C.
   A social history of the minor tranquilizers : the quest for small comfort in the age of anxiety / Mickey C. Smith.
      p.   cm.
   Rev. ed. of: Small comfort. 1985.
   Includes bibliographical references and index.
   ISBN 1-56024-142-X (pbk.)
   1. Tranquilizing drugs—History. 2. Tranquilizing drugs—Social aspects. I. Smith, Mickey C. Small comfort. II. Title. Title.
RM333.S66   1991
362.29′9—dc20
                                                                    91-13143
                                                                          CIP

ACKNOWLEDGMENTS

Although the work on this book spanned several years, the five-month sabbatical granted by the University of Mississippi was critical to its completion. For this I thank Harvey Lewis, then vice chancellor, Dean Wallace Guess, and Robert Freeman, who took the chair in my absence.

James Harvey Young and Glenn Sonnedecker provided tips from their perspective as professional historians and provided the even more important encouragement to continue. John Kallir gave me the flavor of the early advertising, and I was fortunate enough to visit with Leo Sternbach, who not only talked about his work but read the part of my work dealing with his discoveries.

Typing, draft after draft, was supplied by (in alphabetical order) Jean Brannan, Myrna Heimer, Pat Henderson, Frieda McDonald, and Karen Mifflin. Becky Smith provided some original art.

Personal acknowledgment goes to two Dennises, neither of whom would understand how necessary they made the book.

My wife and children have, in this case and always, encouraged without asking too many questions about why. Some time that rightfully belonged to them went into this writing.

Finally, the obligatory but true caveat: Much is owed to those acknowledged above and to others, but they are in no way responsible for errors of omission or commission.

The drug products listed below, and named elsewhere in this book, are the registered trademarks of the companies specified.

Alka Seltzer—Miles Laboratories	Meticorten—Schering-Plough
Alurate—Roche Laboratories	Milpath—Wallace Laboratories
Atarax—T. B. Roerig Company	Milprem—Wallace Laboratories
Ativan—Wyeth Laboratories	Miltown—Wallace Laboratories
Azene—Endo Laboratories	Nardil—Warner—Chilcott
Butisol—McNeil Laboratories	Norlestrin—Parke Davis
Centrax—Parke-Davis	Pathibamate—Lederle
Compazine—Smith, Kline, Beckman	Pathilon—Lederle
Compoz—Jeffrey Martin Company	PMB 200/400—Ayerst
Dalmane—Roche Laboratories	Premarin—Ayerst
Dartal—Searle	Quiactin—Merrell
Darvotran—Eli Lilly and Company	Serax—Wyeth Labs
Decadron—Merck, Sharp and Dohme	Serentil—Boehringer—Ingelheim
Dexedrine—Smith, Kline, and Beckman	SK-Bamate—Smith, Kline, Beckman
Deprol—Wallace Laboratories	Sortran—Stuart
Equanil—Wyeth Laboratories	Soma—Wallace Laboratories
Frenquel—Merrell	Stelazine—Smith, Kline, Beckman
Geritol—J. B. Williams Company	Striatran—Merck, Sharp and Dohme
Libritabs—Roche Laboratories	Suavitil—Merck, Sharp and Dohme
Librium—Roche Laboratories	Thorazine—Smith, Kline, Beckman
Listica—Armour Pharmaceuticals	Trancopal—Winthrop
Meprospan—Wallace Laboratories	Tranxene—Abbott
Meratran—Merrell	Trepidone—Lederle
Meticortelone—Schering-Plough	Valium—Roche Laboratories

CONTENTS

1

PROLOGUE

"The natural role of twentieth century man is anxiety."

Norman Mailer
The Naked and the Dead

In 1982, the Health Research Group of Ralph Nader's organization, Public Citizen, published a 108-page book titled *Stopping Valium*. The book charged, among other things, that

- Thousands of people are addicted to Valium and other benzo-diazepines.
- Many of the 1.5 million people who have taken the drugs continuously for more than four months may be addicted and not know it.
- The drugs present special dangers to the elderly, to pregnant women, and to drivers (Bargman et al. 1982).

In early 1983, it was announced that the recipient of the 1982 John Scott Medal Award for research was Dr. Leo H. Sternbach, the retired Roche chemist who invented Valium and its precursor Librium. Dr. Sternbach was in good company, as previous winners of the award included Madame Curie, Thomas Edison, and James Salk.

How does it happen that a prestigious award is accorded the inventor of substances that a major consumer organization is committed to eliminating? Such an event is, in fact, a typical example of the ambivalence with which our society views the minor tranquilizers. The drugs are more than medicines. They are a social fact. Indeed, these drugs may be more social than medical.

It is the purpose of this book to review the history of this remarkable class of drugs over their first 25 years—from the introduction of meprobamate (as Miltown and Equanil) in 1956 to the beginning of the 1980s.

WHY THIS HISTORY?

Why a history of the minor tranquilizers? Historian Gerald Grob (1977) has presented compelling arguments for the social history of medicine and disease in general.

Grob says that although there is ample evidence that until very recently medical practice had little influence over morbidity and mortality, the response of society to health-related problems has been neglected by historians. This is unfortunate, in Grob's view, as disease is a fundamental part of human affairs. Among its effects are size and structure of the population, living patterns, and technology. Indeed, disease is so basic to existence that the patterns of response to it can tell us much about individual and societal values.

The class of drugs that have come to be known as the minor tranquilizers makes good historical material. Our experience with them is valuable for its own sake, but also for what we can learn from it to apply in the future.

Taking Grob's viewpoint, we might ask whether the period of the 1950s and the 1960s created stress/anxiety, thus requiring drugs to treat them, or whether the availability of the drugs created the conditions.

Branca (1977) suggests that the social history of medicine involves three layers: the great people at the top, the patients at the bottom, and the ordinary practitioner in the middle. Her observations are at least partially applicable to the subject at hand.

"It is necessary," she says, "to look to the hopes and expectations of the patient, and to what doctors had to do to attract patients in order to grasp the development of actual practice, with the top level researcher a necessary precondition for but not always an active cause of change." She takes this line of thought even further, noting that a patient primed for change may jump at innovation, and sometimes "force the ordinary doctor (the intermediary level)—against his will."

Was the patient "primed" for the minor tranquilizers? During the first year of the Reagan administration, *Time* prepared a comparison of the 1950s past and the 1980s to come. Noting that the new tranquilizers of the

1950s (Miltown, Thorazine) saw to the jitters of civilization, *Time* suggested that there were jitters enough to go around. Archibald Macleish is quoted as saying in 1955: "We have entered the Age of Despondency, with the Age of Desperation just around the corner." *Time*'s comment (1981): "Someone is always saying that; it is almost always true."

Do drugs emerge to fit the needs of the times? Burger (1976, p. 26) has noted, regarding the major tranquilizers, "Perhaps the time was right for the discovery of an antipsychotic agent."

With the exception of the oral contraceptives, no class of drugs has the social significance and impact of the minor tranquilizers. Although clearly intended for medical indications, it is just as clear that the medical diagnosis preceding minor tranquilizer use is sometimes imprecise, and further that there has been significant use of the drugs outside of the normal chain of drug prescription and distribution. In spite of the fact that this is the most widely used class of drugs in the world, there appears to be considerable public ambivalence about such use, and recent statistics show a certain degree of decline in use. A similar ambivalence appears to exist in medicine.

In contrast to, for example, antibiotics, whose overuse is opposed on strictly medical (sometimes economic) bases, opposition to use of minor tranquilizers is often couched in social terms, what Klerman (1970) has termed "pharmaceutical Calvinism." Clearly, the minor tranquilizers are a social as well as a medical phenomenon.

New classes of drugs are forecasted that include psychotherapeutic agents to affect memory, learning, perception, and emotions, which will certainly have major social implications. These will bring new challenges that may be better met if we understand the past.

We believe that the minor tranquilizers represent an opportunity to examine the complex interaction between medical innovation and the social structure. These drugs are a fact of our lives, but the reasons for their widespread use have been inadequately explored from either a medical or a social point of view. (Indeed, they have received surprisingly little attention from social scientists). Their use has been questioned on medical, social, legal, economic, even moral grounds, yet this same widespread use indicates an acceptance, perhaps unwilling, by the general public. An understanding of the historical events leading to such acceptance should further our understanding and perhaps even allow prediction of the social and medical response to drugs as yet undiscovered.

In this book, we will argue that the history of the minor tranquilizers is a good example of what sociologists call "cultural lag," which occurs when technological advances outstrip the ability of society to adapt to and to utilize these advances (Stolley 1971). We will suggest that this phenomenon contributes to a therapeutic life cycle for new drug types and will explore some of the social and medical determinants of both the lag and the cycle for the minor tranquilizers.

THERAPEUTIC LIFE CYCLE

The esteemed chemist Alfred Burger has prepared a rich, yet concise history of psychotropic drugs. In it he describes the similar fate of "many new drugs introduced into medicine." An initial greeting, filled with high hopes, is encouraged by science writers and an expectant public waiting for miracles from medicine. Then, Burger says, as tens of thousands of patients are treated with the drug, the known and foreseen cases of side effects are inevitably multiplied until the absolute figures begin to look damaging and the drug may be maligned (Burger 1976, p. 28).

Finally, according to Burger, the medical profession learns to discriminate among patients who should not receive the drug at all and those whose conditions warrant a known and tolerable risk of side effects. At this point, the therapeutic value of the drug (which has not changed) is recognized and the compound finds its appropriate place in therapy.

Does this scenario fit the experience of the minor tranquilizers? At least two serious students of the field have suggested that it does. Sidney Cohen, as a participant in a recent Food and Drug Administration (FDA) committee hearing on the benzodiazepines, described a three-part "law of the new miracle drug":

Part 1. Drugs are overvalued on introduction and soon misused.
Part 2. Problems are discovered and the drugs become undervalued and overcondemned.
Part 3. Stability is achieved with appropriate evaluation of the comparative worth of the drugs (Rickels 1980).

The benzodiazepines, Cohen believed, are still in the second of these stages.

In *The Benzodiazepines*, John Marks agrees that the drugs may be at the low point of the new drug acceptance curve (see Figure 1.1). He suggests that they may be nearing the "rational therapeutic use" point (Marks 1981).

Popular science writer Gene Bylinsky would agree that such a pattern is typical. According to his account (Blinsky 1976), a reading of the mass circulation magazines uncovers the following recurrent pattern:

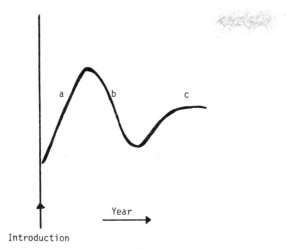

Year

Introduction

FIGURE 1.1 Representation of curve of acceptance for a new drug. (a), Wild enthusiasm, cures everything, no side effects. (b), Nihilism, many side effects, don't use. (c), Rational therapeutic use established. [From Marks, J., "The Benzodiaze-pines—Use and Abuse: Current Status," *Pharmacy International*, Vol. 2, pp. 84–87 (1981). Reprinted with permission.]

- Drug as a curiosity
- Drug as a potential "cure all"
- Dangers of the drug
- Drug as a menace
- Drug as boring

Perhaps the rational therapeutic use of a drug or drug class is boring. There is nothing boring, however, about the kind of roller coaster shown in Figure 1.1, which indicates a period of time, perhaps substantial, during which the actual use of a drug by the population is rarely, and only in passing, equivalent to the putative appropriate use. If there is a way to shorten this process or even eliminate it, perhaps it can be found in history. It is certainly clear that the cycle applies to the minor tranquilizers, as will be discussed in Chapter 4.

CULTURAL LAG

We believe the minor tranquilizers are an example of the cultural lag referred to earlier. Whether they arrived at a time of need or the need was created in response to their availability, it should be clear that our culture has not adapted to and utilized these advances to the general satisfaction of society. They are not unique in this respect. One could argue that the automobile, the computer, and the television set have presented similar knotty cultural problems. In the case of a drug, however, a third party—the physician—is involved. Thus, the patient, the physician, and society as a whole have wrestled together (and too often independently) with identifying the proper role for the minor tranquilizers.

The patient's dilemma has been repeatedly described by the investigators in the only truly national study of tranquilizer use (Manheimer et al. 1973). The researchers concluded that "it appears that Americans believe tranquilizers are effective but have serious doubts about the *morality* [emphasis added] of using them and about their physical safety." In a complete and impossibly difficult twist of reasoning, people had apparently concluded that "moral weakness causes mental illness and taking tranquilizers to correct or ameliorate the condition is further evidence of that weakness."

The physician has problems as well at the interface of the social and the medical. Action oriented, according to sociological studies, the physician is faced with an anxious patient who wants something to be done. Further, given the notoriety of the minor tranquilizers, the patient is likely to know that something can be done. On what basis can the physician withhold antianxiety therapy?

The physician's difficulties have been further complicated by charges both of medicalizing and then treating "problems of daily living." As Freidson (1970, p. 143) has observed: "The medical profession has first claim to jurisdiction over the label of illness and anything to which it may be attached, irrespective of its capacity to deal with it effectively." In fact, people come to physicians because there is anxiety in their lives. By the simple act of seeking medical assistance, the patient has medicalized the problem. Of course, by treating the patient, the physician has confirmed that this medicalization was appropriate. If the drug works, even if only briefly, the actions of both patient and physician are reinforced, and the drugs have worked—criticism of the effectiveness of the benzodiazepines at least has been rare.

Unless and until people are provided with an acceptable alternative to the physician in dealing with their personal problems, as long as they continue to seek relief from this source, it is unrealistic to expect the physician to turn them away because they have a problem with which he or she should not deal. They have come to the physician for help. If the physician eschews treatment (with drugs), the patient is likely to be disappointed (the activism value), and the physician becomes a moral entrepreneur saying, in effect, "You were wrong to come to me. Pull yourself together and get your life in order." However correct that judgment may be, the personal burden on the physician can be enormous.

Unfortunately, the medical professionals charged with administration of the drugs have received surprisingly little assistance from the social scientists who might have offered it. The drugs arrived long before the social scientists were apparently able to deal with them (cultural lag). That is unfortunate, since physicians, especially the general practitioners, might have benefited from the results of sound research on what society expected of these new drugs and the physicians who prescribed them.

With the exception of study in the context of frank drug abuse, which occupied social scientists through the 1960s and into the 1970s, the minor tranquilizers were (and indeed continue to be) largely ignored by sociologists. This can be viewed only as a phenomenal oversight, given their widespread use and social importance.

CONCLUSION

The specific aim of this history is to provide a coherent account of the social, medical, legal, and marketing developments in the approximately 25 years during which minor tranquilizers have been available to the public and to assess the degree of interaction and influence among these developments in this early acceptance and subsequent decline. (The study specifically excludes major tranquilizers, sedatives, and nonprescription tranquilizers, and includes minor tranquilizers, which are defined, for purposes of this study, to include meprobamate, chlordiazepoxide, diazepam, nitrazepam, flurazepam, oxazepam, and chlorazepate, among others.)

This history derives primarily from published information, which is reported both for its own content and to exemplify the information received and (one presumes) used by prescribers, patients, and policymakers in what have become sometimes wrenching medical, social, and even political decisions. The minor tranquilizers are more than medications. They are social facts and artifacts. They are, at the same time, examples of both the power and weakness of medical science.

2

ROOTS

"In the past, we have let ourselves be taken by surprise by the developments of technology. I don't think it was necessary."

Aldous Huxley

DEFINING ANXIETY

The history of the minor tranquilizers cannot be understood without some discussion of the conditions that they treat and the prevalence of these conditions in society. A comprehensive, technical treatment of the subject is beyond the scope of this book and is unnecessary. Nevertheless, a brief examination of some of the issues should be helpful. One of these issues is the elemental one of defining anxiety.

Hollister (1973) has briefly compared the theories of anxiety:

- Cannon (the most popular)—Anxiety is perceived as a threat from within, triggering somatic and visceral responses.
- James Lange—Anxiety is perceived only after the somatic/visceral responses have occurred.
- Freud—Some remembered threat, triggered by something unrecognized in the present, recalls and revives the feeling and somatic responses of the past fearful state.

The title of this chapter can have a double meaning, in that *Rauwolfia serpentina*, the source of one of the basic psychotropic drugs, reserpine, derives its name from the serpentine appearance of the plant root.

- Hughlings Jackson—Mental and somatic aspects coincide closely in time.

Hollister notes that defining anxiety is not easy, but he does distinguish it from fear and tension. He says that fear is acute, with real and recognized causes and immediate, dramatic physiologic responses. Anxiety is more likely to be chronic, its cause ill defined, and its predominant feeling, apprehension, ranging from mildly unpleasant and often resulting in increased effort to paralyzing, totally unproductive mental anguish. Tension, too, is different from anxiety, the latter being purely subjective and the former offering objective signs.

The subjectivity described by Hollister is one of the nagging problems in both the medical and social evaluation of the role of the minor tranquilizers. Mechanic (1978a) provides the sociological perspective, in which the physician's role "is not to decide who is sick and who is not, but rather to be helpful in dealing with a problem once it has been *so defined by the patient and others*" [emphasis added]. Physicians, then, generally assume illness of some kind. Their role is to identify and classify the problem so that they can take some useful action. (The possibility that drug advertising may "help" physicians in identification and classification is examined elsewhere.)

ROOTS OF ANXIETY

What are the origins of anxiety, the etiology? Tessler and Mechanic (1978) examined the relationship between various measures of psychological distress and perceived health status in four diverse samples. In spite of admitted problems of comparison, the authors concluded that there is a clear association between psychological distress and perceived health status, an association that is almost certainly reciprocal. It seems very likely that such causality as it exists may run in either direction. No matter. As Tessler and Mechanic point out, the consistent association between distress and health perceptions further shows that patients experience physical symptoms and dysfunctions in response to their total sense of well-being: "Their notions of physical health both affect and are affected by their sense of psychological vitality." (The effects of the minor tranquilizers on this relationship have not been thoroughly explored.)

The question of whether a certain level of anxiety is normal, perhaps even necessary, is an unanswered part of the criticism of the use of minor tranquilizers.

Rosenfeld (1979) quotes studies showing that some anxiety may be necessary, the so-called "Work of Worrying." He notes Gaylin's suggestion that vague, unfocused feelings of anxiety should be turned into worry, which usually centers on a specific problem or concern about which something may be done: "A healthy anxiety, dealing with things as they are and applying imagination to things as they might become, can lead us to hope and even cheer."

Do the minor tranquilizers, then, hinder this essential self-realization? Opinions pro and con have been expressed, but scientific support for either is obviously difficult to generate. *Time* (1981), in a discussion of the stress experienced by air traffic controllers, asked: "Just how stressful is a controller's job? The short answer: very, but by no means uniquely. The long answer: stress may be what makes a job, and perhaps the people who hold it, a bit more interesting than most."

If, as many have argued, some anxiety is necessary for human existence, the question becomes, How much is too much? If, as del Giudice (1978, p. 140) suggests, anxiety is pathologic when it interferes with moderately optimal functioning, then is not the presence of the anxious patient in the office evidence of pathology?

Clearly, a great deal of stress/anxiety is found in the physician's office. In the 1980 National Ambulatory Medical Care Survey, more than 15 million office visits for mental problems were reported.

But what is a mental disorder?

Again, the sociologist's view sounds a bit nonmedical, although the blurring of the distinction between social and medical was to become an issue in minor tranquilizer use. In any case, sociologist David Mechanic (1978a) quoted estimates that many ambulatory patients (perhaps as high as 50 percent) and many psychiatric patients have complaints that do not fit, respectively, the International Classification of Disease and clearly defined psychiatric syndromes. Instead, Mechanic said, "many of the patients in both populations have a variety of *problems of living* [emphasis added] where classification as disease does little to promote effective treatment."

A further problem is the considerable imbalance between males and females, both in rates of diagnosis of mental conditions and in treatment with psychotropic drugs.

There are difficulties associated with the assessment of rates of mental illness in society, but it appears to be generally accepted that women have measurably higher rates of anxiety and neurosis, or at least report more symptoms. Riessman (1979) has noted that whether this greater reporting is due to clinical status or to sex role prescription regarding acceptable modes for expressing distress has not been resolved. Interestingly, when Riessman set out to determine whether status of the interviewer affected symptom reporting, she found that women reported significantly fewer symptoms to identified physician interviewers (than to lay interviewers), whereas men reported more. This would seem to argue that female data may be underreported.

Radloff and Rae (1979) have suggested that the sex difference in depression, which is well documented, may be due to a sex difference in susceptibility, in precipitating factors, or in both. In any case, the degree to which depression is misdiagnosed as some form of anxiety must be a factor in the sex differences found in the use of anxiolytic agents. In addition to individual differences, diagnosis, and treatment, the mental health picture is further clouded by changing public attitudes.

Jalali and associates (1969) are among those who have tackled the significant problem of public attitudes toward mental illness. They note the two schools of thought: (1) the community mental health movement, which claims that education has resulted in public attitudes that treat mental illness like any other illness; and (2) the "social labeling" model, which views mental illness as a form of deviant behavior that is due to the actions of others and attributes the cause of mental illness to the ascribed social role.

The place of anxiety in either of these two models is not clear. One can hardly label a condition "deviant" that results in the degree of drug use that anxiety appears to. Indeed, one may question (and some data seem to support this) whether the public views anxiety as illness (mental or otherwise) at all.

There is also the apparently widely held public belief that anxiety is somehow a product of and unique to "the times." Rosenfeld (1979), in an intelligent appraisal of the role of scientific "progress" as an anxiety inducer, asked the question: "How much of [our anxiety] can be attributed to the accelerated acquisition of scientific knowledge and its widespread application?" His answer, "Plenty." But not all of it.

Rosenfeld cites Copernicus and Galileo for showing us that we are not the center of the universe, Darwin et al. for identifying us as latecomers to the planet, Einstein for finding new dimensions, Heisenberg for demonstrating the ubiquitousness of uncertainty, Freud and progeny for uncovering our "messy unconscious." Then there are the more tangible: nuclear warfare, ozone-destroying aerosols, cancer-producing foodstuffs, etc.

THE FIRST TRANQUILIZERS

One thing is clear: The availability of effective psychotropic drugs administered by the medical establishment is a recent phenomenon. Wolpert (1968) has noted that as late as 1956 the term "psychopharmacy" was still absent from leading medical dictionaries. The arrival of these psychotropic agents was treated with a curious ambivalence by the medical profession responsible for their administration.

In her fascinating account of the origins of psychopharmacology, Ann Caldwell (1970) identified 1954 as the year in which "modern" psychopharmacology began in Western society. The historical event that triggered this beginning was the first use of chlorpromazine. It is true that psychopharmacologic agents existed already, but as Caldwell points out, "it was [chlorpromazine] that pulled these older drugs from the psychiatric horizon, or even from oblivion." Caldwell further states that "it was [chlorpromazine] that stimulated the synthesis of new drugs, or the use of old ones that existed without ever being used in therapy, like meprobamate, impramime, promazine, and others."

Whether chlorpromazine was, in fact, the strong catalyst described by Caldwell or merely the fortunate first shot in a therapeutic revolution that would have occurred in any case need not be resolved here. It is clear that chlorpromazine and reserpine together formed the basis for new public awareness and hope for real relief from and not just chemical control of mental illness.

Chlorpromazine was followed very closely (in April 1955) by the first compound of a group of drugs that were to become known as "minor" tranquilizers. That compound, meprobamate, under its best-known trade name, Miltown, was to become the best-known drug of its kind, at least for a time.

Less than five years after the introduction of meprobamate, the first of a new class of minor tranquilizers was approved for marketing. Chlordiazepoxide (Librium) seems certain to have achieved a similarly widespread public awareness had it not been eclipsed three years later (in 1963) by one of its analogues—diazepam (Valium). By the mid-1970s, Valium had achieved a level of public recognition and use such that the trade name was used almost generically to mean tranquilizer.

In an article published in the *American Journal of Psychiatry* in 1968, Fleischman very articulately summarized the entry of psychoactive drugs into the mental institution as the "third revolution" in psychiatry (after Pinel and Freud) and also (perhaps unconsciously) anticipated some reactions of the 1970s. As Fleischman put it, the major tranquilizers worked, despite the "sophisticated pessimism" of psychiatrists. In the mental institutions, "delusions and hallucinations decreased, and the understandability and predictability of patients increased. In short, patients became people, and even more important, they become identified as people by the people who took care of them."

Fleischman went on to decry the failure of psychiatry to clearly identify the "third revolution." He asked, "Is it because as psychotherapists, that is, as people accustomed to using words and verbal insights as a means of inducing improvement in the sick, we have a quasi-religious revulsion against the pill?" [This theme was one that would later be expanded and named, by Klerman (1970), "pharmacological Calvinism."]

NAMING THE NEW DRUGS

A substantial literature has sprung up around the issues of classification of psychotropic drugs. The obstacles to a satisfactory classification, according to Shepherd (1972), arose from ignorance about both the drugs and the illness. He noted that disease is usually defined in terms of "etiology," "structure," and "symptomatology," but in most mental disorders etiology is unknown. The structure of the organs of the patients is unaffected, and symptomatology is the only available basis for the definition.

Gerard (1957), reporting on the dozen or so major 1966 conferences on the psychotropic drugs, illustrated the novelty of the area by a preoccupation with names. Pointing out that phrenotropic was "non-committal" (perhaps the reason for its ultimate disuse), *psychotomimetic* was descriptive, and tranquilizer referred only to lessened stimulation, he pointed out that names are *needed* for communication but they carry overtones. Calling a drug a tranquilizer may affect its prescription, the evaluation of its effects, and the label of the patient.

Burger (1976, p. 13) provides interesting background to the terminology that had to be invented. He notes that an early term suggested by Delay, "psycholeptics," was replaced by the term "neuroleptics" to describe the early major tranquilizers. He observed further that the widely used description "antipsychotic" was introduced by a psychiatrist, F. M. Forrest, in a chlorpromazine study in 1954–55. Researcher Howard Fabing and a professor of classics, Alister Cameron, apparently combined to produce the widely used terms "ataractic/ataraxic" (from the Greek noun ataraxia, or calmness), the "ataraktein" (to keep calm), and "ataraktos" (undisturbed). All of these terms are usually, but not always, reserved for the major tranquilizers. The minor tranquilizers are betimes known as anxiolytics and antineurotic and antianxiety agents.

Shepherd (1972) has suggested that the most influential early attempt to subdivide drugs in terms of their therapeutic effects was Cullen's *A Treatise of the Materia Medica* in 1798. He acknowledged Lewin's 1931 attempt at categorizing those "agents capable of effecting a modification of the cerebral functions, and used to obtain at will agreeable sensations of excitement or peace of mind."

Lewins' suggested categories were the following:

1. Euphoriants: "sedatives of mental activity"
2. Phantastica: "hallucinating substances"
3. Inebriantia: substances inducing "a primary phase of cerebral excitation . . . followed by a state of depression which may eventually lead to complete temporary suppression of the function"
4. Hypnotica: "sleep producing agents"
5. Excitantia: "mental stimulants"

Shepard discussed the Delay Classification and noted that it formed the basis for the World Health Organization provisional classification (see Tables 2.1 and 2.2).

Finally, Burger (1976 p. 14) may have identified an important distinction between "drugs" and "medicines." The former (coffee, alcohol, tobacco) might possess a therapeutic potential, but are seldom used in therapy. In contrast, he observed, "true psychopharmacological agents [have] little effect on normal individuals."

PROBLEMS OF DEFINITION AND DIAGNOSIS

According to Dunn (1981), the term "anxiety" has generally been applied to a cluster of symptoms related to the subjective experience of fear, the source of which is largely unrecognized by an individual or which is substantially out of proportion to an actual external threat.

The most prominent classification system is the *Diagnostic and Statistical Manual of Mental Disorders* (third edition) published by the American Psychiatric Association (1980). Despite efforts at classification, however, one medical observer has noted the irony in the fact that anxiety neurosis, the most common indication for benzodiazepine therapy, is the disorder for which their clinical efficacy is most difficult to demonstrate (Greenblatt and Shader 1974c).

A major conference was convened in late 1976 by Medicine in the Public Interest, Inc., to study "the current state of the art of psychiatric practice." One of the 22 conclusions of that conference was the following: "The distinction between major mental illness and 'problem in living' or 'unhappiness' is clear. Evidence is mounting that the most severe and disabling mental illnesses (schizophrenia and the affective diseases) require a pathophysiologic biological substrate for their expression" (Miller 1979, p. 3).

Anxiety can also result in a variety of somatic symptoms that in turn

TABLE 2.1 Delay's Classification of Psychotropic Drugs*

		Examples
A.	Psycholeptics	
	1. Hypnotics acting on mental tonus ("nooleptics")	Barbiturates Nonbarbiturate hypnotics
	2. Neuroleptics acting on mood ("thymoleptics")	Phenothiazines Reserpine and its congeners Butyrophenones
	3. Tranquilizers	Procalmadiol Methaminediazepoxide
B.	Psychoanaleptics	
	1. Stimulants of mental tonus ("nooanaleptics")	Amphetamines and their derivatives
	2. Mood stimulants ("thymoanaleptics") Antidepressives	Diazepines Monoamine oxidase inhibitors
C.	Psychodysleptics	
	Hallucinogenic or oneirogenic substances	Mescaline Lysergic acid diethylamide Psilocybin

*Translated from Deniker (1966).
Source: Shepherd, M., "The Classification of Psychotropic Drugs," *Psychological Medicine*, Vol. 2, pp. 96–110 (1972). Reprinted with permission.

may result in misdiagnosis. Also, anxiety can be secondary to some other functional, psychiatric, or organic disorder. Thus, many prescriptions for antianxiety agents are issued for patients whose primary diagnosis is a somatic disorder (Dunn 1981).

Using data from 50,000 medical patients to whom the Minnesota Multiphasic Personality Inventory was administered, Swenson (1981) showed substantially different profiles for patients with such diverse conditions as pain, nausea, obesity, and rheumatoid arthritis and concluded that "one must at least entertain the hypothesis that, indeed, *all* illnesses

TABLE 2.2 Classification of Psychotropic Drugs Recommended by Special Committee of the World Health Organization, 1967

Category	Representative Members
Neuroleptics	a. Phenothiazines
	b. Butyrophenones
	c. Thioxanthenes
	d. Reserpine derivatives, benzoquinolizines
Anxiolytic sedatives	a. Meprobamate and derivatives
	b. Diazepoxides
	c. Barbiturates
Antidepressants	a. Monoamine oxidase (MAO) inhibitors
	b. Imipramine and other tricyclic compounds
Psychostimulants	a. Amphetamine, methylphenidate, pipradrol
	b. Caffeine
Psychodysleptics (hallucinogens)	a. Lysergic acid diethylamide (LSD)
	b. Mescaline
	c. Psilocybin
	d. Dimethyltryptophan (DMT)
	e. Cannabis (marijuana, hashish, etc.)

Source: Shepherd, M., "The Classification of Psychotropic Drugs," *Psychological Medicine*, Vol. 2, pp. 96–110 (1972). Reprinted with permission.

may be psychosomatic." Eastwood and Trevelyan (1972), in a reasonably well-controlled study, found an intimate relationship between physical and psychiatric disorders and suggested that the usual distinction between the two should no longer be so strongly drawn, but rather pulled together as "manifestations of ill-health of the organism."

Evidence of the far-reaching consequences of anxiety was provided by Howie and Bigg (1980) who used a ten-year retrospective study of the consultations of 50 physicians with a city general practice to test the hypothesis that mothers who receive an excess of psychotropic drugs have children who receive an excess of antibiotics for episodes of acute respiratory illness. The children of the ten mothers classed as high psychotropic users were seen twice as often with acute respiratory illness and received twice as many antibiotics as the children of mothers who had received no psychotropic medication. The association between high psychotropic and high antibiotic use was not linked in time, and indeed the time of highest antibiotic use coincided with the time when the mother received fewest psychotropic prescriptions. It was suggested that at many of these consultations the mother rather than the child should have been treated as the patient.

Medical attitudes toward psychotropic drugs and the conditions they treat have tended to change over time.

In early 1958, Himwich, writing in *Science*, wrote that the new tranquilizers (mostly the major ones at that time)

> may aid in the production of a desirable change in our culture and remove mental disease from the field of mysticism and superstition. They may convince the public that mental disease is not a thing to be ashamed of and that it would be placed in the same category as any other disease which can be treated by medical means.

He noted that the term "psychopharmacologic drug" had advantages, "for it indicates a medicine which influences the *mind* by affecting its morphologic substrate, the *brain*."

Even then, Himwich suggested the use of tranquilizers for "a businessman with a demanding and unreasonable supervisor or a woman with insufficient funds to run her home according to her ideal standard." It should be noted that the suggested use was to render the patient more receptive to other kinds of therapy.

Winkelman (1975), however, took exception to the term "minor tranquilizer" as suggesting that nonpsychiatric disorders are minor psychiatric problems. It would be difficult, Winkelman noted, to tell a patient who has a disabling phobia or obsessive neurosis, who is unable to function occupationally, socially, or sexually, and who is in terror most of the time because of irrational fears and obsessional thoughts, that he or she is suffering from a minor disorder. He argued against drug treatment of the anxiety associated with general living, and was unwilling to accpet a role for "the times" as a causative agent:

> Much has been written about our "age of anxiety" and the stress of our times, although it is likely that each period in history does offer its own stress. Anxious concern about many aspects of society is necessary for normal growth, development, and participation in contemporary affairs. Therefore, unless anxiety is clearly pathological, neuroleptics and anxiety drugs are contra-indicated. (Winkelman 1975, p. 164)

Over the years, as concern over the use of the minor tranquilizers mounted, efforts were made to provide prescribing guidelines to physicians, especially nonpsychiatrically trained general practitioners. But they were rather long in coming.

In a two-part article appearing in the *New England Journal of Medicine* in 1974, Greenblatt and Shader provided "guidelines for the rational use of benzodiazepines in clinical practice." They noted the higher cost of benzodiazepines than of meprobamate and barbiturates, but pointed out that the latter two were also less effective, had a greater abuse liability, and were more likely to produce serious poisoning when overdoses were taken (Greenblatt and Shader 1974d,e).

These suggestions, however valuable, appeared many years after the drugs were introduced.

PROBLEMS OF CLINICAL RESEARCH

How does one measure anxiety, and how does one measure the effect of a medication in reducing anxiety? Those are questions that have plagued researchers from even before the advent of the minor tranquilizers.

In the early 1970s, Hollister (1973a) reviewed some of the clinical research on the minor tranquilizers and noted that in spite of their widespread and continuing use, several well-designed controlled studies had failed to show consistent differences between drug and placebo therapy of anxiety, and observed, rather cynically, that

> the initial treatment used is often efficacious, regardless of what it is .... Anxiety can be a symptom, a concomitant of other physical illnesses, an illness in its own right, or associated with other more severe disturbances such as depression, alcoholism, and schizophrenia. . . . If we are to measure anxiety, we are pretty much at the mercy of what patients tell us. . . . Ordinarily, self-report scales are quite suitable for the predominant symptoms of anxiety . . . but progressively less reliable in depression or psychosis.

Hollister explained the difficulty in measuring improvement in anxiety that might be a symptom, might be associated with somatic illness, might be an illness in its own right, or might be associated with other mental conditions such as depression or schizophrenia.

He highlighted the difficulty in clinical tests for antianxiety agents. It is not that there is a shortage of anxious patients. On the contrary, they are there in abundance, but few are uncontaminated by previous drug use, psychotherapy, concurrent somatic problems, and/or personal problems. Thus, "negative bias" may exist that makes it "almost unrealistic to expect [patients] to show appreciable responses to drugs."

Hollister pointed out the importance of existing test procedures in the drug discovery process, noting that many of the animal tests used for antianxiety agents employ the "barbiturate model." Because of this, he expressed the opinion that a truly different type of antianxiety drug would be unlikely to survive preclinical screening. For this reason, all drugs effective against anxiety at the time of Hollister's observations (1973) were central nervous system depressants.

Finally, one should not overlook the basic principle that studies of the effects of these drugs are simultaneously studies of the workings of the brain and mind. As Berger (1978, p. 14) has observed:

> Psychopharmacology can be defined as a scientific discipline that utilizes drugs to increase our knowledge and understanding of the workings of the mind. . . . Its basic purpose is to help disease, but not to change the personality, improve human nature, or cure bad habits.

CONCLUSION

The minor tranquilizers seem to have been doomed to controversy. There were problems with defining anxiety as well as diagnosing it. Even a name for the new class of drugs was a problem—one that has not been resolved completely. Perhaps the biggest area of controversy, however, has been and continues to be the role in our society of both anxiety and the medications that treat it.

In any case, the drugs are here. In Chapter 3 we shall see how that came to be.

3

DISCOVERY

"Biological psychiatry is an important part of the growing technology for controlling human behavior. To some this is cause for cheering, but to others the future is fraught with terrors for man."

Frank Ayd

EARLY DEVELOPMENTS

The minor tranquilizers sprang from the 1950s, a decade of enormous activity in the pharmaceutical industry. Almost certainly, no other ten-year period in history has seen so many new chemical entities introduced into medical therapy. Not that they were all good. Some were marketing failures, some were medical failures. After all, it was not necessary, during this period, to prove that a drug worked in order to obtain FDA approval.

The psychoactive drugs were but one of several therapeutic classes (antibiotics were another) to achieve their first significance during this period. But they were important. And their beginnings are worth remembering, for such rapid development and marketing are unlikely ever to be seen again.

Caldwell (1978) has divided the history of the development of psychopharmacology into five phases, as follows:

1952-74. This phase was monopolized by the use of chlorpromazine in all mental diseases. It changed the development of sleep therapy and, because of its ataractic properties, made early psychotherapy possible.

Especially important in its impact on society was its effect on mental hospitalization—in both length and character.

1954–57. This was a "boom time" for new tranquilizers. In addition to a variety of phenothiazines, reserpine was introduced to therapy. This period saw the introduction of the first tricyclic antidepressant, imipramine, as well as two new stimulants, methylphenidate and pipradol. The first anxioolytic, meprobamate, which had been synthesized in 1950, reached the market in 1955.

1958–63. According to Caldwell, "Psychopharmacology became the empire Psychotropia! A World Power" (1978). Among the reasons was the growing knowledge of structure-activity relationships and the recognition that therapeutic efficacy and the ability to induce extrapyramidal symptoms were not correlated. In addition to a number of new major tranquilizers, this period saw the synthesis, by Leo H. Sternbach, of chlordiazepoxide (Librium) and diazepam (Valium).

1964–69. Long-acting neuroleptics, a major advance in reducing recidivism among patients, were developed during this period. A number of new minor tranquilizers also appeared.

1970–77. This phase saw the growth of community psychiatry, in large part due to drug advances. At the same time, misuse of some drugs began to bring psychopharmacology some negative criticism.

Caldwell (1970) has argued that clorpromazine stimulated the synthesis of new (psychotropic) drugs or the use of old ones that existed without even being used in therapy. The most important effect of chlorpromazine was to start a new science that gave the old term "psychopharmacology" its true meaning.

Caldwell's historical review of psychopharmacology "from CPZ to LSD" is one of the few book-length accounts of the drug discovery process in the field of mental illness. Others have provided shorter, but nonetheless revealing, stories.

Blackwell (1970), for example, gave a fascinating account of his eventual discovery of the linkage between consumption of certain cheeses (and their constituent amino acids) and the development of hypertensive crises under treatment with monoamine oxidase-inhibiting drugs. Although Blackwell was clearly on the road to this discovery, the process was measurably shortened when his letter to the *Lancet*, noting a fairly frequent association between use of the drugs and hypertension, was read by pharmacist G. E. F. Rowe. Rowe's wife had experienced such episodes twice after eating cheese.

Could there be a link? Blackwell and his colleagues thought not, but a drug "detailman" remembered similar reports to his company. Study and experimentation followed, with results that were certainly lifesaving.

In the same article, Blackwell offered a review of and his own insights into the literature of research creativity. These observations provide an interesting perspective on "the interactions of serendipity, cryptamnesia and adumbration in discovery."

Burger (1976) has prepared an excellent chemical history of the tranquilizers and some philosophical observations as well: "A new science usually emerges from ideas and hypotheses that have waited at low key and spring into full significance when a unifying observation illuminates their background potential." The psychiatric scene was almost totally unprepared for the new drugs, according to Burger. In fact, chlorpromazine and related compounds were first tested as antihistamines. Tests in war showed them to have neurolytic activity.

Burger refers to Janssen's (haloperidol) research skills combined with "the stamina and business acumen to bring this long-range and initially uncertain medicinal gamble to fruition." The parallel to Berger's meprobamate cannot be ignored (see below). He describes the independent works of Berger and Randall in the discovery of minor tranquilizer effects as worthy of study as "lessons in value of an open mind and the need for an encyclopedic knowledge of animal physiology."

THE ROAD TO MILTOWN

Berger's ultimate work on meprobamate started in the 1940s when he was searching for new antibacterial agents as a pharmacologist for the British Drug House in London. It began with the observation of flaccid paralysis of the somatic muscles of mice when injected with α-phenyl-glyceryl ether and some of its congeners. This was not a new observation. It had been known for 36 years, but awaited the push by Berger for the row of dominoes to begin to fall (Burger 1976).

Berger began confirming the α-phenylglyceryl ether work using mephenesin. Animal studies ultimately completed showed a calming effect even at doses that did not lead to muscle relaxation. But mephenesin had problems, related mainly to metabolism, and molecular modification was indicated. In the late 1940s, this work, now being done at Wallace Laboratories by J. D. Ludwig and staff, resulted in a compound, 2-methyl-2-n-propyl-1,3-propanediol dicarbamate, which Berger elected to study in depth. Eureka! It was orally active, lasted eight times longer than mephenesin and was ultimately marketed (and still is) under the name of Miltown, the New Jersey community where Berger lived and where the Wallace Laboratory was located. The approved "generic name" was meprobamate.

Berger (1970) himself has provided a fascinating account of his discovery of meprobamate as well as his own concept of anxiety, its biological basis, measurement, and meaning. He tells us that meprobamate resulted from a "determined and systematic" effort to produce a compound superior to mephenesin. He admits that his work (which took 11 years from the discovery of mephenesin to the marketing of Miltown) was not aimed at the development of either a muscle relaxant or a tranquilizer. Indeed, it was the observation of the muscle-relaxing properties of compounds being treated for toxicity in the search for antibacterial agents that triggered his interest. (A paralyzing effect of a compound closely related to mephenesin had been reported 35 years earlier.)

Berger's attempts to improve on mephenesin continued for years as did his collaboration with B. J. Ludwig, whose contributions he called "all-important." Berger describes in chemical detail the process by which 2-methyl-2-n-propyl-1,3-propanediol dicarbamate (meprobamate) was determined to be the best of the many compounds synthesized. Meprobamate was found to have a duration of action some eight times longer than that of mephenesin and to possess an unusual kind of muscle-relaxant and sedative action. According to Berger, "It also had a taming effect. Monkeys after having been fed meprobamate lost their viciousness and could be more easily handled."

In contrast to most modern drug researchers in the corporate setting, Berger was active in the promotion of this new drug as well as the concept of use of tranquilizing agents. His views were summed up in his own words some 15 years after the marketing of Miltown:

> Koestler has aptly pointed out in "The Ghost in the Machine" that it would be wrong and naive to expect drugs to endow the mind with new insights, philosophic wisdom, or creative power. These things cannot be provided by pills or injections. Drugs can, however, eliminate obstructions and blockages that impede the proper use of the brain. Tranquilizers, by attenuating the disruptive influence of anxiety on the mind, open the way to a better and more coordinated use of the existing gifts. By doing this, they are adding to happiness, human achievement, and the dignity of man. (Berger 1970)

"FIGHTING MICE AND TAME MONKEYS"— THE LIBRIUM STORY

According to Berger (and history), the benzodiazepines were a product of an atmosphere of commercial competition. Irwin Cohen, one of the early clinical investigators of chlordiazepoxide, has stated that the development of the benzodiazepines has never been widely identified with specific persons. (One can argue this point.) He says that "the benzodiazepine story is essentially a model of how a therapeutic agent is conceived and brought forth by an enterprising pharmaceutical manufacturer who simply seeks to find a drug superior to others already in the marketplace" (Cohen 1970).

In fact, the benzodiazepine story, especially Librium, is a good deal more interesting than that. Leo Sternbach has published his own account of the discovery of Librium (Sternbach 1972). His story includes the intelligence that the discovery resulted from a direct search "for new types of tranquilizers." In spite of this specific research agenda, however, serendipity played a hand. Sternbach's full account offers a fascinating insight into the drug discovery process, and is recommended reading, but a verbatim extract is essential here. It begins at a point where corporate research direction and the simple exigencies of laboratory organization meet.

> At that time [this was the second half of 1955] we had to stop our work in the quinazoline field since other problems seemed to be of greater importance. We became involved with other synthetic projects and the isolation, purification, and degradation of various antibiotics. This intensive work, of little practical value, finally led, in April 1957, to an almost hopeless situation. The laboratory benches were covered with dishes, flasks, and beakers—all containing various samples and mother liquors. The working area had shrunk almost to zero, and a major spring cleaning was in order.
>
> During this cleanup operation, my co-worker, Earl Reeder, drew my attention to a few hundred milligrams of two products, a nicely crystalline base and its hydrochloride. Both the base, which had been prepared by treating the quinazoline N-oxide 11 with methylamine, and its hydrochloride had been made sometime in 1955. The products were not submitted for pharmacological testing at that time because of our involvement with other problems. Since the compounds were pure and had the expected composition, we submitted the water-soluble salt for pharmacological evaluation in 1957. We again expected to receive negative pharmacological results and thought that our work with quinazoline N-oxides would be finished and lead to the publication of some chemically interesting material. Little did we know that this was the start of a program which would keep us busy for many years. [Reprinted with permission from Sternbach, L., "The Benzodiazepine Story," *Journal of Medicinal Chemistry*, Vol. 22, pp. 1–7 (1979). Copyright 1979 by American Chemical Society.]

There were chemical surprises in the process as Sternbach describes it, beginning his search with the benzheptoxdiazines, compounds with which he had become acquainted in the 1930s in connection with his studies in dye-stuff chemistry. First attempts at molecule modification aimed at producing desired pharmacologic effects were unrewarding (Sternbach 1972).

Ultimately a compound was produced that did have both pronounced activity and low toxicity—the researchers' "golden fleece" (see Figure 3.1).

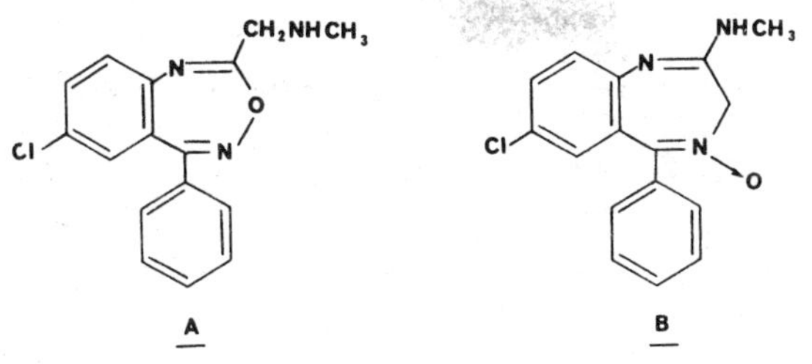

A   B

FIGURE 3.1 The "real" Valium.

The compound was assigned structure "A," while the pharmacological work proceeded. The chemistry of the compound and its starting materials was intensively studied with what Sternbach calls "quite startling" results. First, the chemical structure of the starting materials was not of the benzheptoxidiazines. Second, the reaction that was believed to have produced compound "A" had in fact produced compound "B." This compound, chemically named "methyaminodiazepoxide," and later named, generically, "chlordiazepoxide," was, and is, Librium. The benzodiazepine era had begun.*

Librium, too, was the product of scientific collaboration. In this case, the major collaborator was Lowell Randall, a pharmacologist. Indeed, Hoffman-La-Roche President Clark was later to describe Randall as the "discoverer" of Librium during comments on television's "Sixty Minutes."

Randall (1961), in his early review paper, described chlordiazepoxide as having "unique taming effects in animals and powerful anti-anxiety effects in human subjects." (Note the similarity to Berger's report.) He also described anticonvulsant, muscle-relaxant, sedative, and appetite-stimulating effects. In another paper, he characterized Librium as "qualitatively

---

*One must wonder how Leo Sternbach would react to the following description of the Librium story: "Leo Sternbach stared at the beige walls in Lab 303, trying to invent the scheme that would keep his bosses off his back." B. D. Colen, writing a syndicated column for the *Washington Post*, described it that way. What's more, Colen's account of the discovery is certainly at odds with others. Colen suggests that Sternbach developed compound 0609 at Roche during a period when he was under directions to work on antibiotics, then waited six months before submitting the chemical for fear of "how management would react when they found out he had ignored their orders." According to Colen's account (1980b), Sternbach reported that the compound had been "found" (Colen's quotes) when it was time to clean up the lab.

similar to meprobamate as a tranquilizer, but it is more potent and in addition has taming, and appetite stimulating effects" (Randall et al. 1960).

According to Randall (1961), the difference between chlordiazepoxide and other tranquilizers was noted during the "fighting mouse" test. In this test, pairs of mice are stimulated to fight by application of electroshock to their feet. Most tranquilizers abolished the fighting episodes, but only chlordiazepoxide did so both below the muscle-relaxant dose and without hypnotic effects.

Similarly, chlordiazepoxide demonstrated a "powerful and unique" taming effect in monkeys and, in contrast to other tranquilizers, did so at doses only one-tenth as large as the dose that caused ataxia and sedation. The effectiveness in taming was later demonstrated in tigers, lions, dingo dogs, and squirrels. Valium, which was to follow close on the heals of Librium, was reported by Randall to be "qualitatively similar" but five times more potent (Randall et al. 1961).

A brief chronology of the Librium story would include the following dates:

1930s—Sternbach working on benzheptoxdiazines in Cracow
1955—Reactivation of studies at Roche
1957 (May)—Chlordiazepoxide submitted to pharmacology
1957 (June)—First published data showing muscle-relaxant effect and antistrychnine and spiral reflex blocking
1958 (May)—Patent application filed
1960 (February)—Librium marketed
1960 (March)—First glowing clinical report on Librium in the *Journal of the American Medical Association*

The interval between early pharmacology and marketing was, of course, incredibly short by today's standards. The lengthening time required for this process today is certainly a function of stricter FDA requirements, but equally certainly of the knowledge gained (and subsequently more elaborate testing) as a result of years of experience in the development of psychotropic drugs.

An interesting footnote to the Librium/Valium story is suggested by Temin (1980) in his book, *Taking Your Medicine*. Temin states that the decline in the rate of new drug introductions in the early 1960s was concentrated almost entirely in central nervous system drugs, and within that class in tranquilizers. He suggests two reasons: the thalidomide disaster, which may have discouraged introduction of similar drugs, and the (undocumented) possibility that Roche patented many chemical analogues that might have become competition for Librium and Valium. A number of other benzodiazepines did, of course, ultimately reach the marketplace.

THE SEARCH FOR CLINICAL EFFECTS

The search for drug effects can range rather far afield; in one study, pigeons were taught to stand in a certain position for periods of time with foods as the reward. Use of chlorpromazine was shown to increase the length of time the pigeon was able to sustain the position (Blough 1958). Such a procedure can hardly be used in humans, however, and clinical research on the minor tranquilizers has been fraught with difficulty, frustration, and criticism.

The difficulties in drug evaluation were illustrated by a study of Hesbacher et al. (1970) in which treatment setting (clinic versus general practice versus private psychiatric practice) was found to be at least as important as the medication in producing a treatment response. They noted the "paradox" reported in a personal communication from J. Levine that (in 1968 when their paper was written) 78–80 percent of the prescriptions for minor tranquilizers were written for ambulatory patients of general practitioners and internists, whereas these same drugs were previously tested on hospital patients.

The complexities confronting the clinical researcher who attempts to study and define the effects of minor tranquilizers are further illuminated by the work of Rickels et al. (1972). These researchers set out to determine if such nondrug effects as the "warmth" of the doctor and the clinic setting affected response for drugs under study. They found measurable "warmth" and clinic effects and further found discrepancies with earlier, similar studies.

Newmark (1971) reviewed selective literature of the 1960s concerning psychoactive drug studies. He concluded that "an objective dependent variable is urgently needed which can assess behavioral changes due to drug effects." He further noted that such a measure did not, in 1970, exist.

Even in the early 1970s, researchers such as Samuel Irwin (1972) were calling for a reorientation and redirection of psychopharmacology "from its present trial-and-error empiricism toward a more rational approach."

In 1977, more than 20 years after meprobamate appeared, the FDA, which has ultimate responsibility for evaluating the clinical effects of antianxiety agents, finally published a 16-page set of Guidelines for the Clinical Evaluation of Antianxiety Drugs. It was a bit late in coming.

4

PRESCRIBING AND UTILIZATION

"A trend is not necessarily fate."
Paul Starr
*The Social Transformation of
American Medicine*

Surely a major reason for the controversy that has surrounded the minor tranquilizers, almost from the moment meprobamate was released, was the extraordinary success of the drugs in terms of sales. Much of the criticism has focused not on whether the drugs are safe and effective (although the safety issue has been prominent), but rather on the number of people using them. It is at least possible that some of this concern stems from the extraordinary number of published papers that have expressed dismay about use levels in the abstract, often giving little or no attention to whether such use was appropriate.

Several themes have consistently been used in criticizing the level of utilization of the minor tranquilizers:

1. They do not "cure" anything. (Certainly this is true, but neither does insulin "cure" diabetes nor diuretics "cure" hypertension.)
2. Physicians, encouraged by drug company promotion, have tended to "medicalize" what are basic human problems. This "medical model" has resulted in drug use when social and psychological (nondrug) intervention would have been more appropriate. (Probably true, again, at least in part, but those nondrug alternatives were and are in scarce supply.)
3. Women tend to be overmedicated compared with men, and may be the victim of stereotyping in both diagnosis and treatment. (Also probably true, but with extenuating circumstances.)

28

In this chapter, we will chronicle some of the history of the criticism of minor tranquilizer prescribing and use, review the evidence on utilization, and examine some of the reasons given for prescribing rates.

A report released by the FDA in 1981 indicated that the top prescription drug product for 1980 was Valium. It indicated further that another benzodiazepine, Dalmane, ranked number 11 (Anon. 1981c). In contrast, the National Center of Health Statistics reported that Valium ranked number 10 and Dalmane number 59 among drugs used in office-based practice in the same year (Koch 1982). Which is correct? Elsewhere in its report the FDA cautioned that "there may be several possible answers to any broad question of drug utilization." Indeed!

In 1982, Cooperstock and Parnell published a review of selected studies of psychotropic drug use in England, Canada, western Europe, and the United States. They agreed with Bellantuomo et al. (1980) who had said that "the use of benzodiazepines is perhaps more than a medical practice, as it has probably reached the stage of a mass cultural phenomenon." They also, however, reviewed the methods most frequently used to study the extent and patterns of psychotropic drug use and found each to have some disadvantages. Their comments serve as a helpful reference point in evaluating studies reported later in this chapter.

Every major method of measuring both utilization and prescribing patterns has significant disadvantages. Use of any of the methods such as crude sales data, prescriptions dispensed through various third-party programs or through pharmacies, surveys, or institutional records suffers some problems of over-, under-, or misrepresenting the true picture. This danger has not, however, prevented frequent citation in medical papers of utilization figures in authoritative terms far beyond the quality of the data. Indeed, ongoing, national, reasonably representative data on drug use are available only through commercial sources. The major source is IMS America.

IMS DATA

Although various studies of utilization and prescription rates are reviewed elsewhere in this chapter, none covers the entire 25-year period that began the era of the minor tranquilizers. Indeed, it appears impossible to gather and present such data. Nevertheless, information is available from a single source, using essentially the same methods for much of that time.

IMS America, Inc., is the largest of the pharmaceutical market research firms. It gathers and offers for sale a variety of data on prescribing and promotional activities, among which is the National Prescription

Audit. National Prescription Audit data come from a panel of statistically selected pharmacies across the country and are based as new and refill prescriptions dispensed. These data have served as a basis for FDA estimates of drug use and have been used by other investigators as well. They were used in the estimates presented in this section.*

There are, of course, a multitude of methods of presenting data on these minor tranquilizers. We have chosen just a few in order to provide profiles, both of overall trends and of market behavior.

In Table 4.1, we have continued the data presented by Balter in the early 1970s showing prescription trends for the major classes of psycho-therapeutic drugs. These data show inter alia

- Decline in total prescriptions beginning in 1974.
- Decline in the use of antipsychotics beginning in 1975.
- Dramatic decline in the use of antianxiety agents beginning in 1976.
- Steady increase in antidepressants, which stabilized in about 1976.
- Dramatic decline in the use of stimulants beginning in 1972.
- Slight decline in the use of sedatives over the entire period.
- Decline in the use of hypnotics beginning in 1975.

These same data are graphically displayed in Figure 4.1, whereas in Figure 4.2 the data are shown as a percentage of the total psychotropic drug market held by each drug class at five-year intervals.

It is possible to provide further detail concerning the minor tran-quilizers. Figure 4.3 is an example and shows the market shares of various drugs and drug classes at five-year intervals. Several trends are obvious:

- The growth of benzodiazepines from a 25 percent share (Librium) in 1960 to more than 80 percent in 1980.
- The growth of Valium at the expense of primarily Librium and the meprobamates.
- The effect of the introduction of new benzodiazepines at the expense of Librium and Valium.
- The rather dramatic decline in the meprobamates.
- The stability of the market share for Atarax and Vistaril.
- The growth of generic meprobamates.
- The virtual disappearance, by 1965, of all minor tranquilizers other than the benzodiazepines, meprobamates, and hydroxyzine.

Though not shown here, the sales history of Equanil and Miltown

---

*Although the figures presented in this section were supplied by IMS, the calculations were made by the author. Any errors in calculation and/or interpretation are therefore his responsibility.

TABLE 4.1. Psychotherapeutic Drugs: Prescriptions (in Millions) Filled in U.S. Drugstores, 1964–80

Drug Class	1964	1965	1966	1967	1968	1969	1970	1971	1972
Antipsychotics	14.3	14.8	16.9	16.5	17.8	20.2	21.9	22.2	23.2
Antianxiety agents	45.1	51.7	58.8	59.7	67.8	77.4	83.2	89.1	95.1
Antidepressants	9.5	9.8	12.8	14.8	16.3	19.1	19.8	23.1	25.0
Stimulants	26.7	28.0	26.1	26.8	27.2	26.9	28.2	21.3	11.6
Sedatives	24.1	25.0	23.8	22.4	22.1	22.2	23.8	22.5	20.7
Hypnotics	29.4	31.8	35.7	33.4	33.8	35.9	37.5	39.6	38.7
Total*	149.2	161.0	173.9	173.6	185.1	202.1	214.4	217.8	214.5

31

TABLE 4.1 (continued)

Drug Class	1973	1974	1975	1976	1977	1978	1979	1980
Antipsychotics	23.8	25.4	24.1	22.2	20.1	18.8	18.3	18.0
Antianxiety agents	104.5	102.4	103.2	96.8	90.0	81.1	75.1	71.4
Antidepressants	28.5	32.3	33.0	31.9	30.9	29.5	29.4	29.9
Stimulants	8.6	6.5	6.8	6.6	4.9	4.3	3.3	2.4
Sedatives	20.3	20.0	20.2	19.8	19.3	18.3	18.0	17.3
Hypnotics	37.5	29.4	25.7	21.8	18.4	16.6	14.5	13.8
Total*	223.2	216.0	213.0	191.1	183.6	168.6	158.6	152.8

*Columns may not add up because of rounding.

Source: National Prescription Audit, IMS America Ltd. Drugs have been reclassified and original data reorganized by Balter and associates, Psychopharmacology Research Branch, National Institute of Mental Health, for years 1964–73 (Balter 1975). Data for subsequent years developed from IMS data by present author.

32

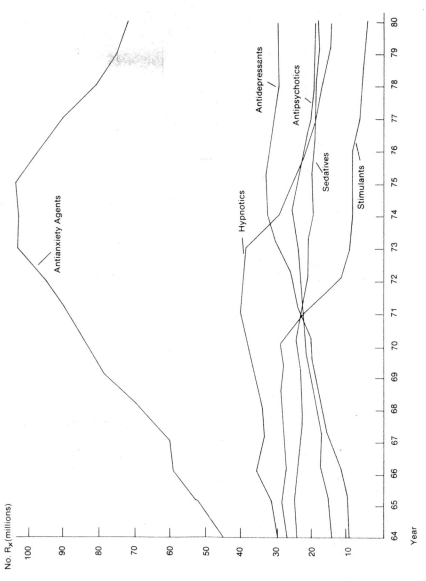

FIGURE 4.1. Prescriptions by class and year. [*Source*: Balter (1975) for 1964–73 data; then IMS America data.]

33

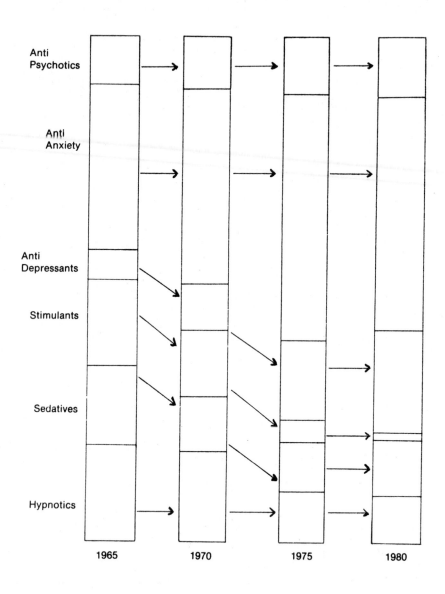

FIGURE 4.2. Share of psychotropic market by class. [*Source*: National Prescription Audit, IMS America Ltd.]

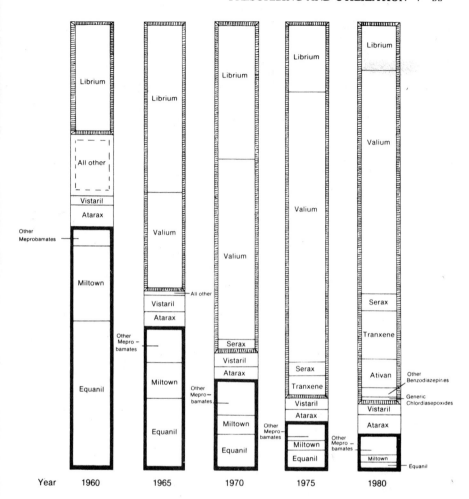

FIGURE 4.3. Share of minor tranquilizer market by drug. [*Source*: National Prescription Audit, IMS America Ltd.]

shows a nearly continuous decline from 1959 when data were first available. In both cases, this decline is, in a major way, a function of the decline in the proportion of refill prescriptions—in the case of Miltown markedly so.

Both Librium and Valium were characterized by a period of several years of steady growth. For both of these products, the decline in total prescriptions was also influenced by a decline in refills in about 1973 (see Figure 4.4 for Valium trends) presumably caused by "scheduling" (see Chapter 9).

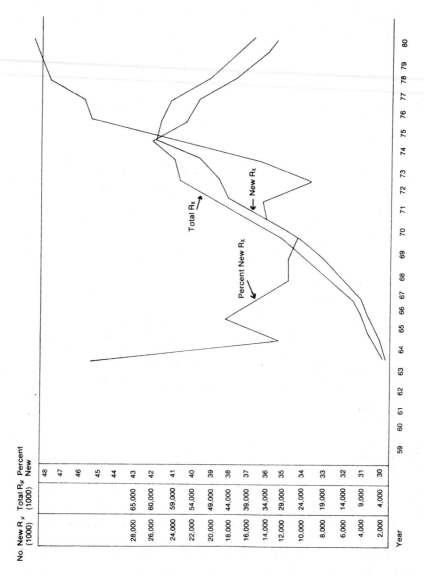

FIGURE 4.4. Valium prescriptions. [*Source*: National Prescription Audit, IMS Data Ltd.]

PRESCRIBING STUDIES

A number of studies of prescribing patterns for psychotropic drugs have been conducted. Unfortunately, many of these studies failed to distinguish between major and minor tranquilizers, sedatives, antidepressants, and other drugs. Consequently, comparisons are often difficult. In this section, we will review chronologically the reports of some of the studies. Some will be reported only in tabular form and a few will not be covered. Included will be several investigations of the reasons for psychotropic drug prescriptions.

Shapiro and Baron (1961) were among the first to study the prescription of psychotropic drugs in a noninstitutionalized population. Their study was conducted in 11 of the 32 medical groups that then participated in the Health Insurance Plan of Greater New York. Even then, the data showed women receiving more psychotropic drugs at more than twice the rate of men. This class of drugs represented 12 percent of all prescriptions studied. Of all psychotropic drugs prescribed, 22 percent were minor tranquilizers. A notable finding, even in this early work, was that only one-third of the prescriptions for minor tranquilizers were written for diagnoses of mental, psychoneurotic, and personality disorders. The percentage so prescribed for all psychotropic drugs was only 18 percent.

A little more than a year later, Baron and Fisher (1952) published the results of a similar study, this time among members of the Group Health Association of Washington, D.C. In this study, minor tranquilizers constituted just over 50 percent of psychotropic drug prescriptions. A striking finding was the fact that "psychological and psychophysiological" symptoms were being treated in only 27 percent of those instances where a psychopharmacological agent was prescribed.

Why do some psychiatrists prescribe drug therapy for their patients more than others? That was the question posed by Klerman (1960) early in the tranquilizer era. Specifically, he tested the hypothesis that the degree of drug use was related to the degree of "authoritarianism" of the psychiatrist and found such a relationship in this study of one mental hospital. The confirmation of this link, suggested by others, was enriched by discussion of some potential implications of the findings. For example, the author constructed a summary of the treatment orientations and value preferences of the study group with the higher rate of drug use.

The psychiatrists in this group, to a greater extent than their colleagues in the "low" group, were found to value assertiveness, self-control, and forceful leadership. Holding these values, they were willing to assume a moderate degree of authority and to exercise their medical responsibility in treating and caring for their patients. According to Klerman (1960), "They consider it their obligation as physicians to use every reasonable means to promote symptom-reduction, to relieve the patient's distress, and to maintain a relatively stable ward atmosphere."

Such attempts at insight into physician drug-prescribing behavior have been extremely rare, and it should be noted that this study did not focus on minor tranquilizers.

Hayman and Ditman (1966) reported on a study (among psychiatrists in southern California) aimed at assessing the relationship between drug use and physician age and theoretical orientation (classical psychoanalysis versus "general psychiatry"). General psychiatrists reported a higher rate of drug use in every type of diagnosis studied.

Some interesting results emerged relative to the minor tranquilizers. The two groups of psychiatrists stated which drugs they used most frequently. When prescribing a "tranquilizer," the general psychiatrists showed a preference for the phenothiazines (major), whereas the psychoanalysts tended to use drugs such as meprobamate or chlordiazepoxide (minor).

Interestingly, when respondents were asked to name the three drugs they used most frequently under each of the following four headings, "Tranquilizers," "Antidepressants," "Antianxiety agents," and "Sedatives," there was considerable overlapping of compounds, illustrating the degree of confusion regarding the meaning of these terms. As an example, six drugs were named in all four categories, and two drugs were named in three categories.

In the early 1970s, Stolley et al. collected some 200,000 prescriptions via a computer in a Pennsylvania community and found psychotropic drugs to account for 17 percent of total prescriptions. Librium and Valium ranked first and third in this study (Stolley et al. 1972). About the same time, Maronde et al. (1969) demonstrated the utility of computer checks on drug utilization. In a study of nearly 53,000 prescriptions, they found that 13 percent were prescribed in excessive quantities, with sedatives and tranquilizers leading the list. These same two classes of drugs also were most frequently involved in situations of concurrent prescriptions with potential interactions on potentiation.

In a related study, Maronde and Silverman (1971) reported significant numbers of prescriptions for minor tranquilizers to be above previously approved limits (e.g., 600 tablets of Valium annually). Some of this was a consequence of patients seeing multiple physicians.

Linn in two related papers (Linn 1971; Linn and Davis 1972) examined attitudes of a sample of 235 Los Angeles physicians toward use of Librium in certain situations. Physicians' general attitudes toward the use of medications were ascertained on the basis of their agreement with the following four statements:

Statement	Percent Agreeing
1. Certain medications are often very helpful in handling	79

the social demands and stresses of everyday living.

2. A person should take pills only as a last resort.	17
3. A person is better off taking a sedative than missing a good night's sleep.	45
4. A person is better off taking a tranquilizer than going through the day tense and nervous.	57

Physicians in the sample were then asked to respond to a number of situations in which Librium was used. As a group, they were not in agreement over what constitutes legitimate use of the drug (see Table 4.2).

In the companion publication, Linn and Davis (1972) added data on physicians' preferred sources of drug information. They reported that physicians preferring professional sources were significantly more likely to express conservative attitudes toward when drugs should be used than

TABLE 4.2. Physician Evaluations of Legitimate Use of Librium from a Medical Point of View (n = 114)

Drug-Using Situation	Assessment of Legitimacy (%)	
A middle-aged housewife having marital trouble takes 15 mg of Librium daily to settle her nerves.	Very Legitimate	34
	Somewhat Legitimate	53
	Not Very Legitimate	7
	Illegitimate	6
		100
A college student takes 15 mg of Librium occasionally when the stresses and demands of college life become too great.	Very Legitimate	20
	Somewhat Legitimate	41
	Not Very Legitimate	21
	Illegitimate	18
		100
A physician takes 15 mg of Librium occasionally when the stresses and demands of his practice become overbearing.	Very Legitimate	17
	Somewhat Legitimate	38
	Not Very Legitimate	25
	Illegitimate	18
		100
A college student, highly anxious, takes 15 mg of Librium daily to combat anxiety.	Very Legitimate	22
	Somewhat Legitimate	31
	Not Very Legitimate	25
	Illegitimate	22
		100

Source: Linn, L., "Physician Characteristics and Attitudes Toward Legitimate Use of Psychotherapeutic Drugs," *Journal of Health and Social Behavior*, Vol. 12, pp. 132–139 (1971). Reprinted with permission.

physicians preferring commercial sources and were significantly less likely to feel that medical advice from sources other than a physician was acceptable. Linn and Davis suggested that the medical profession contains "rather diverse philosophies of medication."

In an unusual study, Vaillant and associates (1970) had the opportunity to study the use of mood-altering drugs by 45 physicians who had been involved 30 years earlier in a study of the psychological health of college sophomores. Eighteen percent of the physicians reported using tranquilizers regularly, compared with 7 percent of a control group (n = 59) consisting of nonphysicians from the same study population. The authors found that one-third of the total time the group of physicians had spent in the hospital had been the result of self-medication with drugs or alcohol. They concluded, "No physician, whatever his rationalization, should write a prescription for himself for a drug that will make his brain feel better, sleep better, or work better."

Parish (1973) reviewed the factors involved in the increased prescribing of psychotherapeutic drugs and gave much of the credit (or blame) to influence by the drug industry, although he noted that perhaps inadequate training of general practitioners to deal with emotional problems was a factor as well. That was just about the time that utilization began to decline, but the change had hardly been noticed.

Hollister (1973a) stated that same year: "It is uncertain whether this increase [in the use of antianxiety agents] is the result of the generally turbulent times which have prevailed in the past decade, or of the introduction of new drugs and their widespread promotion, or of sloppy prescribing practices of physicians." He suggested five reasons for the extensive popularity of the benzodiazepines in comparison with meprobamate or barbiturates:

1. They are virtually "suicide proof."
2. Metabolic tolerance is less; i.e., they are less likely to lose their clinical effects.
3. The duration of action is longer than that of meprobamate, resulting in the need for less frequent dosage and in sustained clinical benefits.
4. They are poor candidates for physical dependence (although Hollister himself showed as early as 1961 that physical dependence with chlordiazepoxide could occur).
5. They produce remarkably little change in normal sleep patterns.

Others were not so sure. Mayfield and Morrison (1973) had reviewed all outpatient prescriptions for minor tranquilizers for the calendar year 1970 at the Durham (North Carolina) Veterans Administration Hospital. Their conclusions were among the harshest rendered by physicians in a medical journal. They stated in their abstract:

> This study reveals a significant indictment of what is widespread practice—the misuse of the minor tranquilizers. On the basis of otherwise highly satisfactory records, it is obvious that the use of tranquilizers was without rhyme or reason. Without doubt this represents common practice—a pill because a patient wishes a pill—without thought as to drug dependency or untoward side effects. The rational use of drug therapy of whatever kind demands knowledge of its pharmacologic effects.

They concluded:

> Characteristically physicians in their use of ataractic drugs: do no make observations of behavioral features relevant to drug therapy; do not organize their observations into a clinical condition; do not select the type of drug, amount and schedule of administration on an informed rational basis; and do not follow the course of treatment by making observations of treatment-relevant factors to be compared with pretreatment status. (Mayfield and Morrison 1973)

Reports began to appear with frequency citing "high" rates of psychotropic drug prescribing (Rosenberg et al. 1974; Skegg et al. 1977). Often they included opinions about the quality of that prescribing.

Ingman et al. (1975) studied prescribing and administration of drugs for 131 patients in a nursing home. They found that prescriptions written "PRN" resulted in more drugs being administered than were prescribed. They also found that "neuroactive" drugs were used more often for patients with higher mental status and physical independence. Minor tranquilizers were prescribed for 19.8 percent of the patients. About the same time, Nightingale and colleagues (1975) editorialized that "most inappropriate prescribing is by the well-intentioned physician who is either not fully informed as to the potential effects of his prescribing or who allows himself to be manipulated by persons selling drugs."

Davidson et al. (1975) examined the prescribing habits for psychotropic drugs of internists, surgeons, and gynecologists on their inpatient wards in a teaching hospital. Data were gathered from patients' charts and pharmacy records. In a six-week period, 9 percent of all admissions received such a drug, of which 72 percent were minor tranquilizers. Less than half the available drugs were used, but drugs of different groups were often used interchangeably in an unsystematic fashion. There was little evidence on the chart as to how effective a drug had been. It also seemed that depression was often overlooked or insufficiently treated. As the authors noted, "It seems [the psychotropic drugs] are applied uncritically in many cases, with little recorded either to identify the nature of the disorder they are supposed to treat, or to indicate their effectiveness." In an expansion of that paper, they reported results of interviews with the physicians who did the prescribing. They found that minor tranquilizers were prescribed most frequently "and with least justification" (Raft et al. 1975).

Much of the attention regarding the minor tranquilizers has focused on utilization of the drugs themselves—usually with emphasis on high rates of such utilization. It is rarely suggested that use of these drugs may have an overall salutory effect on medical care utilization. Neither do we suggest such an effect. We do note, however, the important work of Tessler et al. (1976), which showed a positive relationship between psychological distress and physician utilization, even when a variety of sociodemographic, attitudinal, and health status variables were controlled.

The authors' analysis revealed that the effects of stress on utilization were primarily direct, but that some indirect effects were also present and mediated through certain health status variables. They suggested an overall perspective that attributes to distress a "direct causal role," and that emphasizes social psychological needs as "triggers" for physician utilization.

Not all studies were negative. In an interesting and somewhat reassuring study that involved Valium only because of nurses' familiarity with it, Rank and Jacobson (1977) set up an experiment to see if nurses would comply with an apparently legitimate physician's order for an overdose. Sixteen of the eighteen nurses in the study refused to do so, although a previous experiment had achieved the opposite results with a fictional drug. Rickels and Hesbacher reported, in 1977, on a 1970 study of drug use in seven family practices. They concluded that, at least in these cases, prescribing was appropriate, although it was noted that the family practitioners had been trained in clinical research by the authors.

Elena Hemminki's work in Finland was part of the early research on the importance of the use of tranquilizers for somatic conditions. In her study, which unfortunately did not differentiate between minor tranquilizers and other psychotropic drugs, she found one-half of such prescriptions associated with physical ailments.

She also included in her analysis combination products, which included both a psychotropic ingredient and one or more other active ingredients, referring to such products as "hidden psychotropics" (Hemminki 1974a). Hemminiki's discussion for her findings was quite critical:

> Variations may occur in the factors that induce doctors to prescribe psychotropic drugs for somatic diseases. First of all, most of the somatic diseases have a psychic component, either as cause or result. It may be assumed that much of the therapy was directed to the relief of psychic symptoms induced by physical disorders, even though no separate mention was made of the psychic component. Secondly, the psycho-

somatic concept, that much in somatic diseases is a reflection of psychic disturbances, may offer an explanation for the abundant use of psychotropic drugs; the therapy has been no more than of derisory nature. It might be regarded as an expression of incompetence; the doctor, incapable of applying other therapeutical means, prescribes a drug, on this occasion a psychotropic one.

Hemminki gathered data both on physician prescribing patterns and on certain professional attitudes. In the latter case, she used attitudinal statements previously employed by Linn. The more positive the physician's attitude toward the use of drugs for social problems and everyday stress, the more psychotropic drugs were prescribed (Hemminki 1974b).

Williams (1978) has reviewed this use of "mental" drugs for "body" ailments and suggests three kinds of reasons why psychotropic (mainly minor tranquilizer) drugs are prescribed for physical illness:

1. Secondary properties of the drugs. Examples include reserpine in cardiovascular disease and diazepam as a muscle relaxant in arthritis/rheumatism.
2. Coexistence of physical and psychiatric disease. This is purported to be a function of (a) increased likelihood of physical morbidity among the psychiatrically ill; (b) increased likelihood of psychiatric morbidity among the physically ill; (c) existence of some individuals who are prone to both types of illness.
3. Psychic component of somatic disease. (The evidence cited in support of this type of use is reported to be weak.)

It is, of course, more likely that a general practitioner will see the patient with some kind of mind/body problem.

Raynes (1979) used the technique of tape-recorded observations in her study of the interaction between client and general practitioner. In reporting "preliminary findings" in 249 observations, she found that some kind of drug was prescribed in 63.8 percent of the consultations, even though no diagnosis was made in 39.1 percent of them. Analysis of those consultations revealed that a diagnosis of psychiatric disorder was present in 28.1 percent of the psychotropic prescriptions, but psychosocial problems were present 59.5 percent of the time, leading her to suggest that treatment is symptomatically, rather than diagnostically, based.

Much has been made of the fact that general practice physicians treat the majority of the anxiety in the United States. These physicians, of course, have the option of referral for the patients, just as they do for surgery and other "specialty" problems, although psychiatrists are not readily available in some areas. Hull (1979) studied nonpsychiatrist views of psychiatric referral among 93 such physicians in four Chicago communities, two predominantly white and two black.

Hull began by asking about patients attitudes and found substantial consensus that patients are less likely in recent years to be annoyed or frightened by a psychiatric referral, physicians should not hesitate to refer out of concern for labeling the patient a "mental" case, and neither should referral be avoided because patients may believe the physician views their problems as imaginary. Respondents were then queried about their actual referrals. Some two-thirds of the physicians agreed that all cases of psychoses should be referred to psychiatrists, but the remaining one-third covered the entire spectrum of alternatives, indicating that there is lack of a norm for psychiatric referral of psychotic patients.

There was much less consensus about the use of referrals with neuroses. About one-third made no referrals, one-sixth referred all cases, and the remainder again covered the entire spectrum.

Abbott et al. (1983) studied psychiatric diagnosing in a group of family practitioners and found, via multiple-regression analysis, that the patient score on the Cornell index was the only variable significantly associated with such diagnosis. Hypotheses related to social factors such as patient stereotyping were rejected. Drug use was not studied per se.

Near the end of the first 25 years with the minor tranquilizers, T. Donald Rucker (1980), a health economist, essayed a quantitative opinion about the causes of "irrational" prescribing of minor tranquilizers. His estimates, which appear in Table 4.3, reflect rather well the themes that have emerged, though the proportions hardly constitute a consensus.

UTILIZATION STUDIES

In addition to studies of prescribing and prescriptions, some researchers have used the patient as the unit of analysis; i.e., What proportion of a population used the drug under study? Parry (1968) was one of the first to present extensive data on the utilization rates for psychotropic drugs. He commented that this group of drugs had been "generally neglected by social researchers" in favor of the "more exciting, glamorous, and dangerous" hard and psychedelic drugs.

Parry noted that psychotropic drugs accounted for 14 percent of all prescriptions in the period 1963–65 and pointed out that two-thirds of these prescriptions were refills, compared with about 50 percent for other drugs. "The preponderance of refills," Parry wrote, "[tended] to operate against any sharp decline in consumption."

Parry's data came from different sources. The first source was a national sample of adults including nearly 4,000 respondents. They found

TABLE 4.3. Factors Leading to Irrational Prescribing Classified by Quartile of Probable Level of Importance

Proportion of Problem		
50%	I.	Promotional activities sponsored by pharmaceutical manufacturers that are designed, directly or indirectly, to influence practitioner prescribing and dispensing
		Limitations in the medical record system
		Casual empiricism—practitioner interpretation of evidence regarding patient response to drug therapy
About 30%	II.	Drug product proliferation without significant therapeutic contribution
		Practitioner attitude toward treatment options in general, and drug therapy in particular—the subjective component
		Patient behavior—designed to influence prescribing patterns and subvert coordination of care
About 20%	III.	Formal education received by practitioners
		Practitioner postgraduate education [excluding promotional activities identified in (I), but including all other inputs or lack thereof]
		Practitioner proficiency in diagnosis, and selection of optimum modality within treatment model
Nearly 10%	IV.	Various characteristics of practice environment
		Conflict of interest situations
		Posture of professional associations toward drug use and drug industry

Source: Adapted from Rucker (1980).

that 14 percent had used tranquilizers. Examples used in posing the use question included both prescription (Miltown, Librium) and nonprescription (Compoz) drugs. The results of Parry's study as well as others conducted subsequently are shown in Table 4.4.

TABLE 4.4. Increase in Use of Tranquilizers, 1957–67

Surveys and Questions Posed	Date of Survey	Number Surveyed	Percentage Using
American Institute of Public Opinion: "Have you ever heard of pills called tranquilizers? (If YES) Have you ever tried them?"	March 1957	1,550	7
Psychological Corporation: "By the way, have you yourself ever had occasion to take a tranquilizer?" (asked of those who could define word "Tranquilizer")	February 1960	3,885	14
American Institute of Public Opinion: "Have you ever taken a tranquilizer?"	July 1960	1,440	25
Social Research Group	September 1967	3,390	26

Source: Parry, H., "Use of Psychotropic Drugs by U.S. Adults," *Public Health Reports*, Vol. 83, pp. 799–810 (1968). Reprinted with permission.

Parry found higher proportions of use, in broad terms, among women, higher-income groups, and Jews. Data available on the use of alcohol led him to suggest that some of these differences might be attributable to use of the drugs as an alternative to alcohol. Lower-income groups tended to use more nonprescription and fewer prescription drugs. There were also data suggesting some economic class specificity; i.e., the upwardly mobile tended to use drugs in a pattern similar to that of the economic class into which they were moving.

In another primarily methodologic report, Parry and associates (1970–71) assessed the degree to which respondents in studies such as their's might "underreport" the use of psychotropic drugs. Using a population known (from another study) to have had prescriptions filled for such drugs, the researchers conducted interviews among them. They found tranquilizer users to be significantly more likely than users of sedatives or stimulants to give valid responses to questions about such use. About eight of ten correctly stated that they had received tranquilizers.

Manheimer and his associates (1968), in a paper published at about the same time as that by Parry, studied psychotropic drug use by adults in

California. Based on a sample of just over 1,000, the study showed that about 30 percent had used some type of psychotropic drug in the previous 12 months. About one in six used the drugs frequently, with women users outnumbering men by about two to one.

As with many utilization studies, the results are clouded by the combination of several types of psychotropic drugs, both prescription and nonprescription. One interesting finding with regard to use of prescription drugs (particularly tranquilizers) by lower-income groups was that while they were less likely overall to use them, their use, when it occurred, tended to be frequent. Manheimer et al. suggested that only those with substantial need in this group actually get the drugs.

Prevalence of use, however, varied greatly by sex and age of the person, by therapeutic class, and by intended and actual source of drug. Persons between 45 and 59 years old were more likely than others to use prescription drugs from medical sources. Use of over-the-counter drugs and prescription drugs obtained from nonmedical sources was most prevalent among persons aged 18–29. Overall, prevalence of psychotherapeutic drug use was highest among persons under 30 years. Persons who obtained prescription drugs from nonmedical sources were more likely than others to use a variety of drugs, but were less likely to use any drug regularly (Mellinger et al. 1971).

Chambers (1972) has reported on a broad-range study of drug use projected to the population of the state of New York in 1970. Because of the extensiveness of the study, we will offer considerable detail in tabular form. General use levels are shown in Table 4.5, with some specific findings in Table 4.6.

TABLE 4.5. Incidence and Prevalence of Relaxant and Minor Tranquilizer Use*

	Number	*Percentage*
Never used	10,734,000	77.9
Former users (no use in last 6 months)	1,334,000	9.7
Infrequent users (fewer than 6 times per month)	886,000	6.4
Regular users (at least 6 times per month)	525,000	3.8
No data	305,000	2.2
Total	13,784,000	100.0

*Defined as diazepam (Valium), chlorodiazepoxide (Librium), meprobamate (Miltown, Equanil), etc.
Source: Adapted from Chambers (1972).

TABLE 4.6. Specific Findings in New York State, 1970

•70.5%	of regular users are female
•45.0%	of regular users are unemployed females "presumably housewives"
•85.3%	of regular users are white
•88.0%	of regular users secured the drug with a legal prescription
•Significant proportions of regular users use one or more other drugs	

Source: Adapted from Chambers (1972).

Notably, the two largest consumer studies to this point in the chronicle of the drugs were conducted in two of the most cosmopolitan areas. A national study did not appear until the early 1970s. We refer (page 49) to the work as the "Balter" studies although many researchers were involved. Other, smaller-scale utilization studies continued to be conducted.

Zawadski and associates (1978) used the California Medicaid data base to compare the amount of pattern of prescription drug use among the aged with that of the general population and then compared, within the aged population, drug use by the institutionalized and noninstitutionalized. It was found that prescription drug use was higher for the aged as compared with the general population; among the aged, however, prescription drug expenditures were almost three times as high for the institutionalized as compared with the noninstitutionalized. The bulk of the difference in prescription drug expenditure among the aged subgroup was found to be due to a much higher level of psychotropic drug use. One of the most interesting findings of the study was the confirmation of previous research results showing an increase in drug usage with age, but with the further finding that institutional residence was the real factor accounting for these results.

In the Boston Collaborative Study, 25,258 patients were interviewed on admission, 5,079 had taken a psychotropic drug in the prior three months, and 68 percent of these (14 percent of total) took an antianxiety agent. The percentages taking antianxiety agents were diazepam, 45 percent; chlordiazepoxide, 32 percent; barbiturates, 13 percent; and meprobamate, 8 percent. Of those who used them at least once a week, more than half had done so for a year or longer (Greenblatt et al. 1975).

The federal government has not totally ignored the drug use issue. Koch (1982) reported on the 1980 data gleaned from the National Ambulatory Medical Care survey. In these data, Valium ranked as the tenth most frequently used drug (about 1 percent of the drugs mentioned). The next highest ranking minor tranquilizer was Tranxene (no. 58), followed by Atarax (no. 81), Ativan (no. 104), and Librium (no. 116). These five drugs together accounted for about 2 percent of the drug uses reported.

In October 1981, the FDA released what was described as its first annual summary of drug utilization. Data were actually obtained from IMS America and covered the years 1977, 1978, and 1979. In each of those years, benzodiazepine minor tranquilizers were the single largest category of drugs used, as shown below.

Year	Prescriptions (Millions)	Percentage of Top 19 Categories
1977	76.4	11.6
1978	68.4	10.4
1979	62.3	9.7

In December 1982, a similar FDA report, covering the year 1981, showed a 33 percent decline in the use of benzodiazepines for the period 1973–81, although Valium still headed the list of most prescribed single drugs. The difficulty of assessing drug use statistics is shown by a comparison with data from the National Ambulatory Care Study (above).

THE "BALTER" STUDIES

In the first quarter-century of the minor tranquilizers, only one truly national study of utilization was conducted. A number of researchers were involved in this project, which was conducted under joint sponsorship of the National Institute of Mental Health (NIMH), the Social Research Group (George Washington University), and the Institute for Research in Social Behavior (Parry ct al. 1973). The research resulted in a considerable number of publications, some of which contained similar data. Because their's was the only one of this magnitude in the 25-year history of the minor tranquilizers, it deserves special attention. It should be noted that the national survey was, in fact, the culmination of a series of studies begun in 1966.

The work has often been cited by those defending the minor tranquilizers, but, perhaps significantly, rarely attacked by the drugs' various opponents. The principal researchers in this series of studies were usually at pains to avoid "taking sides" in issues over tranquilizer use. They noted some of the problems:

> In too many instances the physician finds himself willy-nilly in the position of adjudicating philosophical and emotional conflicts. It is as if he were suddenly thrust back more than a century and faced with such a nightmare controversy as "Is the Use of Chloroform in Childbirth Against God's Will as Revealed in Scripture?" (Parry et al. 1975)

On the other hand, they were not reluctant to speak from data:

> There is no real evidence that the American People are "over-medicated" with respect to psychotherapeutic drugs, and, in fact, there is considerable evidence that they take them rather sparingly and under physicians' orders; and that many of the users take them with such puritanical reservations and qualms as would have warmed the heart of John Calvin. (Parry et al. 1973)

The comprehensive report of this collaborative study appeared in the *Archives of General Psychiatry* in June 1973 (Parry et al. 1973). The data were based on extensive personal interviews (60–90 minutes each) with 2,552 adults selected through "rigorous probability sampling methods" throughout the 48 contiguous states in late 1970 and early 1971.

As with many other studies, this one included a variety of psychotherapeutic agents. Because of our focus on the minor tranquilizers, and in the interest of space, we list below some of the specific findings based on the survey relative to this class of drugs.

- Most current users felt they were helped by them.
- The percentage using minor tranquilizers/sedatives during the previous year is shown below.

			Age		
	18–29	30–44	45–49	60–74	All
Men	5	7	9	11	8
Women	12	21	22	25	20

		Region		
	Northeast	North Central	South	West
Men	7	7	7	13
Women	18	17	21	25

- Women were more likely than men to say they would take a tranquilizer in advance of a possibly unpleasant event.
- The United States would rank about in the middle of western countries in level of use of minor tranquilizers, and the male-to-female use ratio is similar.
- About 5 percent of users utilized minor tranquilizers daily for at least two months (defined in the study as "high" use).
- Among users whose use level of minor tranquilizers was "high," the following characteristics appeared important:
  1. greater proportion in middle age

2. greater proportion in the west
3. greater proportion in lower socioeconomic class (similar to Parry's findings).
• There was little overlap between prescription and nonprescription tranquilizer use.

Balter has attempted to find some meaning in these data. In his 1973 presentation to the Anglo-American Conference, he reviewed some of the utilization data from the studies of his research group. Among the issues he addressed was the degree to which drug users may have been responding to symptoms and life crises.

We now come to the question of the extent to which persons using psychotherapeutic drugs are emotionally distressed and/or suffering severe or traumatic disruptions in their life situations, particularly those persons who have used psychotherapeutic drugs regularly over extended periods of time. In popular terms, this issue might be best viewed as a question about the degree of provocation, i.e. whether the patient was sufficiently ill or his life situation sufficiently disrupted to justify his visit to the doctor and his treatment with a psychotherapeutic drug. For some persons this is a straightforward clinical question; for others it is more a characterologic or value question about personal or cultural standards of suffering or illness. (Balter 1973)

Using a symptom checklist and the Holmes-Rahe Social Readjustment Scale, it was possible to classify persons in terms of emotional distress and life crises. One of the principal findings was that 60 percent of the men and 70 percent of the women who used psychotherapeutic drugs in the year preceding the interview scored high on one or both indexes, psychic distress, and life crises. Among the relatively small group of persons who used the drugs daily for two months or longer, the figures were somewhat higher: 70 percent of the men and 80 percent of the women.

A majority of the remaining drug users who were not classified as high on one index achieved a rating of at least moderate on the other. Only 2–3 percent of those who used drugs daily for two or more months were classified as low on both indexes, as compared with 16 percent of persons who used no psychotherapeutic drugs in the preceding year.

In the autumn of 1971, Balter and associates obtained data on the use of antianxiety/sedative drugs via a household survey in nine western European countries. As in the United States, women were more likely to have used such drugs by a ratio of two to one. The countries with the highest proportion of respondents reporting use of the drugs in the previous year were Belgium and France (17 percent); the lowest was Spain (10 percent). Little relationship was found overall by country between level of use and attitudes toward the drugs. There were, however, sharp differences between users and nonusers on whether the drugs "do more harm than good," with nonusers more negatively disposed to the drugs (Balter et al. 1974b).

In one paper from the series, based on data obtained in Oakland, California, an attempt was made to relate use of minor tranquilizers and sedatives to the existence of health problems. A clear relationship was found between drug use and the existence of symptoms, mostly psychologic. Only a modest relationship was found, however, between drug use and various indexes of role performance impaired becaue of the existence of symptoms. The authors in their comments noted the following:

> Drug use did not seem differentially related to the presence or absence of situational problems as such, without additional disturbance. These data suggest that the use of minor tranquilizers and sedatives is consistent with a rational medical model in relation to both the type and the amount of disturbance experienced.
>
> There was a modest tendency for minor tranquilizer users to seek concomitantly other possible help as well, including medical care, other prescription medications, and increased use of coffee or tea. Exceptions included the lower use of snacks and alcohol by men and the lower used of over-the-counter nonpsychotropic medications by women. These substances apparently were used largely as alternatives to minor tranquilizers. These data suggest that the use of minor tranquilizers and sedatives is only one element in complex patterns of copying behaviors employed in combination or interchangeably to deal with distress and dysfunction.

Responding to the frequently expressed concerns, they noted:

> To evaluate whether we are an "overmedicated" society would require in addition the application of a value system to the information. It would require weighing not only the desirability of using minor tranquilizers, but also the desirability of the probable alternatives, some of which have been noted above. (Uhlenhuth et al. 1978)

The response to psychic distress and life crises by using psychotherapeutic agents is described in greater detail in a 1978 article in the *Archives of General Psychiatry* (Mellinger et al. 1978). Some of the data are shown in Table 4.7. The authors asserted that their data do not support the contention that these medications are commonly prescribed for persons with minor and transient disturbances of minor consequence.

Mellinger et al., concluding their report on the relationship between psychic distress and drug use, noted the varied criticisms of psychotherapeutic drug prescribing. Taking the many criticisms at face value, they

TABLE 4.7. Relation of Psychic Distress and Life Crisis to Psychotherapeutic Drug Use*

	Any Past Year (%)	Regular (%)	Alcohol Use (%)	Number
Women				
Psychic distress				
Low	12	3	18	560
Medium	20	5	21	425
High	34	14	27	504
Life crisis				
Low	15	4	16	352
Medium	21	7	21	627
High	26	9	27	510
Men				
Psychic distress				
Low	6	3	51	566
Medium	10	3	53	434
High	23	10	60	210
Life crisis				
Low	7	1	42	295
Medium	10	3	53	434
High	13	7	64	310

*Tranquilizers (minor and major), daytime sedatives, and antidepressants. Figures refer to use of drugs obtained through conventional medical channels, excluding hospital use.

Source: Mellinger, G. D., Balter, M. B., Manheimer, D. I., Cisin, I. H., and Parry, H. J., "Psychic Distress, Life Crisis and Use of Psychotherapeutic Medications," *Archives of General Psychiatry*, Vol. 35, pp. 1045–1051 (1978). Reprinted with permission. Copyright 1978, American Medical Association.

observed, "One might well conclude ... that a marked reduction in pharmacotherapy is an intrinsically desirable goal both socially and medically." Noting the ideological and moral character of some criticisms and the difficulty of testing others empirically, they raised a number of questions requiring answers prior to accepting the above-mentioned goal as a self-evident truth.

THE SEARCH FOR CAUSES

Throughout their history, the minor tranquilizers, their use and prescription, have been studied in efforts to determine reasons for their popularity. Some hypotheses have already been noted. Others, resulting mainly from research, are presented in this section.

The use of psychotropic drugs in cases with nonmental diagnoses may have a number of explanations. One of them may be found in studies such as that by Locke and Gardner (1969), who found psychiatric problem rates ranging from 5.2 to 23.4 percent coexisting with medical diagnoses.

Gardner (1971) suggested that broadening the indications for the drugs may account for increased use: "It is only now that we are faced with the possible utilization of psychoactive drugs by a major portion of the population in what might be considered problems of daily living." He noted that there is time to deal with this, but that it is also necessary to do so. Discussion is needed, he suggested, about the desirability of relief or freedom from all psychic pain, and in this sense, whether we want a "drug dependent" society.

In 1970 and 1972, Pflanz and colleagues conducted a survey in Hannover, West Germany, among 1,251 subjects (1977). They found that 14.7 percent of the men and 27.1 percent of the women took tranquilizers "regularly" and "presently." Consumption was higher in the upper and middle classes, particularly for men. They also found a strong relationship between drug consumption and mental health (as assessed on a 22-item scale). Drug use was shown to be related to subjective ill health and unrelated to objective indicators of health status. The researchers saw the data as supporting a psychiatric medical model rather than a sociological one (Pflanz et al. 1977).

This last issue was at the core of the study. Pflanz et al. reviewed the literature of sociological studies of tranquilizer use and found that while a variety of cultural and social variations were reported, the one unanimous finding was a higher rate of use in women—and this finding was not dependent on the respective status of women in the various counties.

In the Pflanz study, some of the findings were the following:

- Users were more "health conscious."
- Homemakers were not found to be heavier users than employed women.
- There was no relationship between drug use and role status inconsistency.
- Some 29 questions about "mental health" distinguished between users and nonusers, which was "true for mainly somatic symptoms, for psychosomatic symptoms, and for purely psychological symptoms" (perhaps most significant).

Pflanz and colleagues made a special effort to isolate the factors involved in the consistently higher use of tranquilizers by women. They found it appropriate to assume that women have more psychological symptoms and therefore take tranquilizers more often than men. They also found support for the hypothesis that women perceive and express more symptoms of ill mental health than do men. They finally raised an interesting reverse question: Is the question why do women take more, or why do men take less? Again, the assumption appears to be that less is better.

Greenblatt and Shader (1974c) were concerned about use levels: "In a three-month period, approximately one in 10 American adults will take diazepam because of tension or nervousness. Symptomatic anxiety is extremely common among the adult population, but whether it is severe or prevalent enough to justify this extent of pharmacotherapy is questionable."

According to Cooperstock and Lennard (1979), the people who are most likely to receive prescriptions for minor tranquilizers fall into three groups:

1. Those who describe their problem to the physician in psychological or social terms.
2. Those who describe physical complaints (insomnia, stomach pains, backache), but who are discovered to experience "problems of living." (For women these tend to relate to structural strains in the nuclear family. For men they are more likely to be job related.)
3. Those with chronic somatic illness for whom the drugs may be prescribed to diminish stress generally and in reaction to the illness particularly.

They noted also that "since the legitimation of a personal problem as a 'disease' affords considerable advantages, it is readily 'traded' for a medical diagnosis."

Publication of such studies culminated in one of the strongest attacks on the increased prescribing of Valium, Librium, and other drugs. Waldron (1977) presented a plethora of arguments (some supported, others not supported) to the effect that these and many other drugs are often prescribed for nonmedical (i.e., social) reasons. She referred to the "extremely rapid" increase in the use of Valium and Librium, referring especially to the advance of Valium, from its introduction in 1963 to the top seller in 1972. (In fact, that is not "rapid" by drug industry standards, and suggests, instead, a steady rise based on positive experiences.)

Waldron noted the use of Valium and Librium in somatic conditions even though "these drugs have not been shown to alleviate hypertension, angina, peptic ulcer, or asthma." Similarly to Hemminki, she used the term "hidden psychotropics" to refer to products containing a minor tranquilizer in combination with other drugs [e.g., meprobamate and tridihexethyl chloride (Pathibamate) for ulcers] and claimed that they represent one in three minor tranquilizer prescriptions.

Quoting drug advertisements for such conditions a major discord in parent-child relations, she noted that they appear

> to offer a resolution for a common and difficult dilemma for doctors, namely, how to respond to a patient who is distressed by psychological and social problems, given that both the doctor and the patient expect the doctor to do something to relieve the patient's distress in an appointment that averages less than twenty minutes. (Waldron 1977)

Such prescribing for social and psychological problems, Waldron noted, "appears to satisfy substantial needs of both doctor and patient." Indeed, even she agreed that the period of increasing use of Valium and Librium was also a period of increasing social problems.

Waldron also argued that the vaunted effect of the major tranquilizers on mental hospital discharges was greatly overstated. Whether her arguments are correct or not, the fact is that many people in the 1950s believed in this relationship and that belief must certainly have contributed to the ultimate acceptance of the minor tranquilizers.*

In the late 1970s, Tessler et al. (1979) concluded a study in Massachusetts in which 5 physicians and 55 pharmacists distributed approximately 800 questionnaires to Valium users in the central and western state. Some 236 were returned and these formed the basis of their report.

They found a two-to-one female-to-male ratio among users, normal physician utilization, reasonably good social contact, and the previous use of other tranquilizers by about 50 percent. Most did not request the drug. Rather it was recommended by their physicians, nearly half of whom gave little or no information about it. Two of five expected beneficial effects, but one-fourth were worried about side effects or dependence.

More than 95 percent felt they had been helped by Valium, but one of three felt it would be either fairly or very difficult to reduce or stop use of the drug. Interestingly, and consistent with other studies, nearly half admitted reservations about the use of tranquilizers, generally on "ethical or moral grounds." Most denied ever recommending use of the drug to others.

---

*One of the difficulties with many of the more harshly critical papers on minor tranquilizer use is the frequent failure of the authors to apply the same rigor to their own arguments that they appear to expect from drug company promotion. Waldron, for example, uses references dealing with drug promotion practices that are not only second or third attributions, but some of which predate the period which she is discussing.

In a community (Washington County, Maryland) survey, Craig and Van Natta (1978) found that 41.8 percent of 771 men and 60.2 percent of 1,054 women reported using one or more medication in the 48 hours prior to the interview. Respondents who used four or more medications tended to score higher on a depression checklist than did those who used fewer drugs.

Perhaps most disturbing was the finding that the group of women who used minor tranquilizers and sedatives included significantly more high-depression scorers than those who did not. Craig and Van Natta clearly suggest that depressed individuals may be inappropriately treated with "non-specific remedies" which "at least offer merely palliative symptomatic relief and, at worst, may intensify the distress they are intended to treat."

It has been hypothesized that in achievement-oriented societies, illness may be used as justification for a culturally induced sense of personal failure to fulfill socially prescribed role obligations. Prince (1978) has produced data that are consistent with this hypothesis, which had been formally proposed by Cole and Lejeune (1972). In a study with admitted limitations of previously hospitalized patients, Prince found that welfare recipients were more likely to consider their health as fair/poor than those not on welfare. Cornely (1978), in a commentary, denounced not only the study itself, but studies of the genre, urging social scientists to study such factors as employment, housing, nutrition, environmental sanitation, and personal accountability.

Other researchers continued to search for determinants of tranquilizer use in a variety of places.

Webb and Collette (1975) examined an hypothesis that urban crowding might be associated with a higher incidence of use of stress-alleviative drugs. They found the reverse relationship and further that such drug use increases directly with the number of persons living alone.

Khavari and Douglass (1980) approached the use of psychotropic drugs in a novel fashion, hypothesizing that drug use is determined by a sort of "cost-benefit" analysis performed by the user. Their methods, which are open to some question, show the minor tranquilizers (which they call "relaxants") between alcohol and amphetamines on their cost-benefit index.

Radelet (1981) set out "to identify health beliefs and social networks that distinguish users from non-users." His population consisted of only 181 university students (46 of whom used tranquilizers), but his findings were interesting. He found the users, in comparison with nonusers, to be

- more reluctant to admit unpleasurable feelings
- more likely to define anxiety as a biophysical problem
- less critical of over-the-counter drug advertisements

- more likely to have friends and relatives who use tranquilizers (especially the father)
- more anxious as measured by Spielberger's State-Trait Anxiety Inventory

Radelet acknowledged that symptoms of anxiety play a role in tranquilizer use, but argued that they are only part of the picture. He wrote, "The extensive prevalence of tranquilizer use in American Society is therefore not indicative simply of high levels of anxiety, but also is associated with a general cultural framework that tends to define anxiety as an individual biophysical reality that warrants and necessitates drug treatment."

There has been speculation that the high rates of psychiatric treatment for women in Western society reflect not only true morbidity but also a greater propensity among women than men to seek professional help for emotional problems. Kessler et al. (1981) presented evidence from four large-scale surveys that documents this role of differential propensity. Although screening scales of psychiatric morbidity in all four surveys showed women to have more emotional problems than men, there was also a consistent tendency for women to seek psychiatric help at a higher rate than men with comparable emotional problems. A decomposition of the help-seeking process into stages showed this sex difference to be due largely to the fact that women translate nonspecific feelings of distress into a conscious recognition that they have an emotional problem more readily than men do. Evidence was presented that between 10 and 28 percent of the excess female psychiatric morbidity measured in treatment statistics could be due to this sex difference in problem recognition.

BALTER'S VIEWS

NIMH researcher Mitchell Balter (1975) has produced some of the most thought-provoking commentary on the utilization of the minor tranquilizers, noting the "widespread belief" that antianxiety drugs are "needlessly and inappropriately prescribed on a large scale." Who is at fault? Balter observes the variously attributed blame—physicians' attitudes, training and knowledge, shortcomings in the system, the avaricious drug industry, or, perhaps most pervasive, moral decay. In fact, Balter's studies show that more than two-thirds of those persons receiving prescriptions for antianxiety drugs actually suffered from a medically significant degree of psychic distress.

Balter has referred to developments in the antianxiety drug market as "drug cannibalism." Thus, meprobamate usurped the market lead of phenobarbital in the late 1950s, only to be passed in the early 1960s by chlordiazepoxide, which in turn was passed by diazepam. But, Balter observes, no matter what drug was in the ascendancy, be it meprobamate, chloridazepoxide, or diazepam, and despite promotional activities that tended to emphasize the differences between the drugs, the overall pattern of use by diagnosis for the class as a whole has remained fairly constant. What emerges is the strong impression that there is a definite place in the general practice of medicine for a safe and effective all-purpose sedative with muscle-relaxant properties, and the drug that best meets those requirements at a particular time is the one that comes to be prescribed most frequently.

Balter presents figures indicative of an increase in the proportion of patients who received an antianxiety or sedative drug from 8 to 12 percent of all patient visits in the period 1964–73. Nevertheless, he points out that the origin of the increase—more persons treated, more chronic use, higher rates of prescribing—is unknown.

Balter (1975) has made an unusual proposal, as yet not implemented, that there be

> a major research effort to determine what public attitudes are and to use the public as an active resource in the development of standards and basic principles just as certain professional organizations have used their membership to develop codes of ethics for research and treatment. . . . In this manner, it is possible to pose classical dilemmas and to gauge public sentiment on some crucial issues of cost, benefit, and risk. [From Balter, M., "Coping with Illness: Choices, Alternatives, and Consequences," in R. Helms, ed., Drug Development and Marketing, Washington, D.C., American Enterprise Institute for Public Policy Research (1975), reprinted with permission.]

In a telling comparison, Balter contrasts official and social views of drug use, on the one hand, for hypertension and, on the other, for anxiety. Quoted here, they argue for perhaps an alternative interpretation of the results of some studies cited in the previous section.

> In the case of hypertension the official position is that drug treatment is both possible and desirable.* This position implies that we know the morbidity and mortality of the disease, that we have effective drugs that can reduce both morbidity and mortality, and that we both know and are willing to accept the consequences of long-term use of these drugs. In the case of psychic disturbances and the antianxiety agents, the sentiment is

---

*Quoting FDA Commissioner Charles Edwards.

to allow the untreated cases to remain untreated and to reduce the number of persons in treatment, on the assumption that most of those seeking treatment do not merit it. Whether these contrasting positions on hypertension and psychic disturbances can be justified on the basis of lifetime morbidity and mortality is open to question. Over the past ten years, evidence has been accumulating that life crisis and stress may be etiological factors in a wide variety of illnesses, but the effects of intervention with psychotropic drugs have yet to be determined.

The crucial point of all of this is that, both as a society and as professionals, we often speak glibly about the overuse of pharmaceuticals without ever having established the true prevalence of the diseases for which the drugs are intended. If by overuse we mean that drugs are being prescribed for the wrong people or for the wrong reasons or that their potential for harm is worrisome, we should say so and then separate these more refined judgments from vague negative generalizations about sheer increases in the volume of prescribing. It is important to remember that better treatment of many diseases and better health care for previously neglected subgroups in the population are quite likely to produce what most people would regard as laudable increases in the overall volume of drug consumption. [From Balter, M., "Coping with Illness: Choices, Alternatives, and Consequences," in R. Helms, ed., *Drug Development and Marketing*, Washington, D.C., American Enterprise Institute for Public Policy Research (1975), reprinted with permission.]

In the late 1960s, Balter and Levine (1969) testified before the Subcommittee on Monopoly of the Senate Select Committee on Small Business. Their testimony was based on early studies of the Special Studies Section of the Psychopharmacology Research Branch of the NIMH. They cited prescription data from commercial sources as well as the 1967 study of the Social Research Group at George Washington University. Among the "somewhat surprising" findings was the use of the minor tranquilizer drugs for mental disorders for only 26–34 percent of the time. Even these early reports noted the "generally conservative" attitudes of the public toward the use of tranquilizing drugs.

Speaking to the Anglo-American Conference on Drug Abuse in London in 1973, Balter noted the heavy social (as opposed to medical) content in critical views of the use of psychotherapeutic drugs:

The evils of psychotherapeutic drug prescribing and use within the medical system is a popular, eminently appealing and salable theme in a society desperately searching for the elusive causes and solutions to the problems of serious drug abuse. The medical system is a ready scapegoat because it lends itself to social control through legislation or regulation—whether the actions are germane or not—whereas the more critical aspects of the illegal traffic in drugs are not directly control lable.

> The issue of psychic illness is particularly sensitive because it lies at the interface of pathological social conditions and personal failure—a very different situation from that of classic organic illnesses.

Balter went on to caricature the popular stereotype of the doctor-patient encounter vis-à-vis psychotherapeutic drugs:

> The ignorant, greedy, indifferent, and irresponsible physician—the simple dupe of the drug industry—shoveling out drugs to the weak, devious, irrational, and highly manipulative patient who is not really sick—he is just feigning illness or is unwilling to tolerate mild discomfort—or who is merely seeking drugs for kicks or trying to escape the unpleasant realities of every day life. In any case, the patient is intent on getting drugs, no matter what.

Balter summarized the issues relating to the rationality or appropriateness of prescribing psychotherapeutic drugs as including such questions as whether it is appropriate to use psychotherapeutic drugs

1. to offset severe pathology in a classic psychiatric disorder.
2. as adjunctive treatment in a psychosomatic disease where there is presumption of underlying stress, e.g., peptic ulcer or hypertension.
3. as symptomatic treatment in a crisis situation of short duration, e.g., accidents, death (grief), divorce, reaction to terminal illness.
4. to improve adequate social functioning in highly demanding situations, e.g., meeting a deadline, driving a long distance, coping with an emergency.
5. to anticipate or offset anxiety or discomfort, e.g., fear of the dentist, fear of flying.

The answers to such questions still await consensus.

COOPERSTOCK ON WOMEN

One social scientist who has devoted a great deal of effort to the study of the use of minor tranquilizers is Ruth Cooperstock of the Addiction Research Foundation in Toronto, Canada. She as much as any other has focused on sex differences in use. In 1978, her review of the literature on the use of these drugs demonstrated that women exceed men in their consumption of psychotropic drugs in a consistent ratio of two to one (1978a). She notes that this suggests a "certain immutability." She observes further, however, that the frequently quoted studies of the Dohrenwends (1974) "showed a consistent pattern over time and place of women reporting more neurotic illness than men and, by contrast, the personality disorders appearing the male prerogative" (Cooperstock 1978a).

As Cooperstock observes, women, in study after study, report more of both emotional and phyical symptoms than do men. Whether these differences that appear in so many studies reflect a greater sensitivity to emotional and bodily reactions on the part of women, i.e., an ability to feel discomfort, or simply a willingness to express discomfort to an interviewer or on a self-report form remains a moot point in her view.

Searching for reasons for the increasing use of minor tranquilizers, especially by women, Cooperstock seems to feel that some can be found in the "expansion of the bounds of medical care" to include a variety of social problems. As Cooperstock observes, "If financial difficulties, loneliness, and disobedient children are commonly seen as problems presented to physicians then we must hardly be surprised by the increase of psychotropic drug consumption that has taken place in the past decade." It is not known when this paper, published in 1978, was written, but certainly there is room for argument that such drug use increased in the decade. "These 'problems of living' have somehow become 'medical problems' by definition, if only because they came up in the physician's office." Further, she notes, the pharmaceutical industry has provided the tools to treat the problem.

Why the difference in male and female use of drugs and reporting of symptoms? Hard answers are not available, although opinions abound. Cooperstock quotes Nathanson (1975), whose review of morbidity studies concluded that employment has, perhaps, the most positive effects on women's health of any variable investigated to date.

Is there a difference in symptoms or in reporting symptoms? The evidence is confusing, but interesting. Coates (1982) reported that even when "perceiving themselves to be on the point of a nervous breakdown, men were only half as likely as women to go for professional help." In another study, this time in New Zealand, the psychotropic drug consumption patterns of single women were found to be similar to those of all adult men (Thompson 1973).

CONCLUSION

The minor tranquilizers are still among the most widely used classes of medication. There has been a proportionate decline in their use since the mid-1970s, when use reached a peak.

Prescribing of the drugs has been roundly criticized, usually for its frequency. There is, however, some evidence that the relationship between diagnosis and treatment is not always clearly drawn in the physician's mind.

There has been and is considerable concomitant use of the drugs with medications used to treat physical ailments. Whether the level of such use is too high (or too low) has not been decided, although opinions on the subject are not scarce.

Women use tranquilizers to a greater extent than men—about twice as much, according to Cooperstock. Though she has provided a logical and appealing model to explain some of the reasons, it is notable that the determinants tend to be social rather than medical.

5

THE ROAD TO MILTOWN—MASS MEDIA COVERAGE

> "He is not acquainted with drugs; and I know that the prevailing impression on his mind is, that Epsom salts means oxalic acid; and syrup of senna, laudanum."
>
> Charles Dickens
> *Pickwick Papers*

When, in 1957, just months after the product reached the market, S. J. Perelman published a book of essays entitled *The Road to Miltown*, nobody had to be told that he was not referring to a small town in New Jersey.†

Miltown specifically and the minor tranquilizers in general have always "enjoyed" a great deal of press coverage. Meprobamate arrived on the scene in the middle of a therapeutic decade that was notable for the public attention given to new drug developments.

Morton Mintz (1965) in his book, *The Therapeutic Nightmare*, included an entire chapter on the subject of media coverage of new drugs. That chapter, entitled "Drug Success = News; Drug Failure = Non-News," was harshly critical of the press reportage of new prescription drug developments. Mintz wrote,

---

A shorter version of this chapter appeared as Smith (1983).

†Interestingly, Miltown's "twin," Equanil, never caught the public fancy in the way the Wallace product did. Equanil did, however, consistently sell better. The fact that Wallace had no sales staff must have been among the reasons, but it is also possible that physicians preferred to prescribe a drug with a less-well-recognized name. One wonders how the history of the drugs might have been altered if Wallace Labs had been located in Newark.

64

The press had exhibited a tendency to regard drug success or *claimed* success, as news, and drug failures as non-news. This has been a highly significant factor in the lack of public awareness that some of the highly touted prescription drugs laymen demand, and get, are ineffective and therefore dangerous.

Mintz suggested that the members of the press were willing collaborators in the indirect promotion of new drugs through planted publicity stories. The so-called "wonder drugs" of the 1950s were unlike their nonprescription predecessors since they could not be advertised to the public. Yet, as Mintz pointed out, "the public hungered for news of wonder drugs that promised to save lives, curb disease and ease pain." What happened, according to Mintz, was the following sequence:

1. Public wants drug news.
2. Reporters look for drug stories.
3. Drug industry "plants stories," often withholding vital facts.
4. Patient, aroused by promises of relief, pressures physician to prescribe new drug.
5. Physician accedes.

Mintz described examples of these practices involving Norlestrin, Decadron, and penicillin. He quoted Dr. Hobart A. Reimann as follows:

Popular magazine articles, television and radio programs, and commercial advertising have glamorized and exaggerated the value of these "wonder drugs." Because of this, lay persons often insist on the treatment or prevention of many ailments for which antimicrobics have no value.

Although Mintz offered considerable criticism of various practices of the marketers of the minor tranquilizers, which were in their ascendancy as he was writing, he did not cite them among examples of inappropriate use of the news media. Nevertheless, this class of drugs was destined to become the most widely prescribed in the history of medicine. Was the popularity due, even in part, to glowing reports in the nation's lay press? Although an absolute answer to that question is an impossibility, we provide here some historical data on the subject.

The materials that were reviewed for this study were articles indexed in the *Reader's Guide to Periodical Literature* for the years 1954–81. It is recognized that this procedure can provide only a partial picture of the information that the public received about these drugs. Radio, television, and newspapers certainly contributed, and still do, to public views of the minor tranquilizers, but a retrospective analysis, at least of the first two of these media, is well-nigh impossible.

The term "tranquilizer" did not appear in the *Reader's Guide* until

1957, with a reference to "see Sedatives." On the other hand, meprobamate had already achieved separate listing.

An amazing amount of publicity accompanied the introduction of the tranquilizers, although public understanding must certainly have suffered from the confusion between the major and the minor tranquilizers, both classes of which appeared in close time sequence. (One suspects some physicians might have been confused as well, and early articles in the medical press bear this out.) Clorpromazine and reserpine paved the way for the public introduction of the minor tranquilizers, and although the present chapter focuses on the latter, it is often difficult to separate the drug classes in press coverage.

The popular writers were faced simultaneously with an opportunity and a problem. The opportunity was, of course, a brand new class of drugs. They affected the mind, in itself somewhat of a mystery, and gave promise of being especially newsworthy.

The problem (which still exists with such new developments as interferon and genetic engineering) was how to make the mechanism of action of the drugs—the technical details—understandable to the average reader. Something was needed to grab the reader's attention and at the same time communicate. What often were used to fulfill these two needs were catchy terms of the type shown in Table 5.1—euphemisms, a little "cute" in some cases, but telling the reader at a glance what to expect from the article.

More than half of the terms in Table 5.1 appeared in the 1950s, when the drugs were new and interest was high. The decline in their use in more recent times resulted, in all probability, from a dearth of new terms and the increasing sophistication of the reader. (After a while, it was logical to start calling tetracycline an "antibiotic" and stop calling it a "wonder drug.")

There were more than catchy terms in the material in the lay periodicals. For many members of the public, these sources were often the first introduction to the minor tranquilizers, or at least their first opportunity to read in-depth reports. Careful reading of what the public read may provide some insight into the response to this unusual sociomedical phenomenon. What follows, then, is a review of the treatment of the minor tranquilizers (primarily) by the lay magazines.

THE 1950S

As noted above, the minor tranquilizers had been foreshadowed by the major tranquilizers. In 1954, for example, *Life* ran a dramatic series of pictures showing a monkey calmed by reserpine and a rat quieted by chlorpromazine, under the headline "Good Medicine from Medicine Man."

TABLE 5.1. Tranquilizer Euphemisms in the Lay Press, 1954–81

Year	Term(s) Used	Source
1954	"Wonder Drug of 1954"	*Time*
1956	"Happy Pills" "Aspirin for the Soul"	*Changing Times*
1956	"Psychiatric Aspirins" "Mental Laxatives"	*Nation*
1956	"Pacifier for the Frustrated and Frenetic" "Don't-Give-A-Damn Pills" "Pills for the Mind"	*Time*
1956	"Peace-of Mind Pills"	*Coronet*
1956	"Happiness Pills" "Emotional Aspirin"	*Newsweek*
1956	"Happy Pills"	*Look*
1956	"Happiness Pills"	*Christian Century*
1957	"Peace of Mind Drugs"	*Today's Health*
1957	"Happiness by Prescription"	*Time*
1959	"Happy Pills"	*Coronet*
1960	"Calming Pills"	*Science News Letter*
1960	"Peace of Mind Drugs"	*Time*
1961	"Quiet Pills"	*Today's Health*
1962	"Turkish Bath in a Tablet"	*Reader's Digest*
1963	"Brain Drugs"	*Popular Science Monthly*
1964	"Mind Drugs"	*Science Digest*
1966	"Weak Barbiturates" "Weak Alcohol"	*Science News*
1966	"Mind-Acting Drugs"	*Science News*
1969	"Psychotropes"	*Transaction*
1980	"Bottled Well-Being"	*Time*

In February of that year, *Science News Letter* (1954b) gave a very positive report on reserpine, and in April (1954a) it issued one of the early reports on chlorpromazine as an effective treatment for severely ill mental patients. Two months later, *Time* (1954) called chlorpromazine the "Wonder Drug of 1954."

Some of the problems with journalistic reporting are illustrated by the *Science Digest* (1955a) headline "'Drugged' Artists Paint Better," a story, mostly negative, of the effects of lipergic acid diethylamide (LDS). In fact, three of the four artists who received the drug had to be coaxed to paint at all!

Time (1955) featured the new psychotropic drugs in a lengthy article, "Pills for the Mind." Only chlorpromazine and reserpine were discussed in an optimistic but objective article. Although calling the drugs "as important in their way, as the germ-killing sulfas discovered in the 1930's," the article also noted that "even the most enthusiastic advocates of the drugs ... emphasize that by themselves the pills and injections probably do not cure anything." (This theme was to be repeated in the lay and medical press for the next quarter-century.)

In July, *Science Digest* (1955b) issued a brief report based on six-month studies of chlorpromazine and reserpine, and quoted Dr. Roy Grinner: "Tranquilizer is the best name for these drugs. They are the best pharmacologic agents to come along since the barbiturates." This was one of the earliest uses of the term "tranquilizer" in the lay press.

Consumer Reports (1955) provided a review of mental disorders and focused on chlorpromazine and reserpine. The verdict—the drugs are valuable but hope for a cure-all for mental illness is premature. Simultaneously, *Cosmopolitan* published one of the first and one of the most glowing reports on Miltown. In a subheadline of the article, it reported: "Safe and quick, Miltown does not deaden or dull the senses, and is not habit forming. It relaxes the muscles, calms the mind, and gives people a renewed ability to enjoy life" (Galton 1955). There must have been joy in Miltown when that appeared. Case studies were presented showing improved sleep and relief from the "blues," stomach distress, neurodermatitis, even excessive perspiration. The author was obviously sold on the product.

> Many attempts have been made to find a method of reducing tension quickly. Of the numerous drugs which have been tried, Miltown comes the closest to being ideal. It relaxes muscles; it calms the mind; it blocks undesirable nerve action; and it accomplishes its overall tranquilizing effect without deadening or dulling the senses. The case histories of many patients testify to its effectiveness. (Galton 1955)

The next year, still failing to differentiate between major and minor tranquilizers, *Changing Times* (1956) said Americans "have in the past couple of years taken to gulping pills to make them happy." Calling them "happy pills" and "aspirin for the soul," the article made clear the benefits of the drugs, but suggested that the same agents that had such salutory results in institutions were tried on 20–30 million "psychoneurotics who are not ill enough to be hospitalized but who suffer agonies from obessive fears and psychosomatic ailments." (Such use would have included as many of 20 percent of the population.)

Earlier, H. Azima (1956a), a lecturer at McGill University, was coining terms for the *Nation*: "psychiatric 'aspirins'," "mental laxatives" (to purge people of "noxious spiritual alimentations"). In his somewhat negative review ("A critical pedantry may be preferable sometimes to vulgarized falsity"), he examined two major and two minor tranquilizers (meprobamate and azacyclonol).

Azima described Azacyclonal (Frenquel) as "the least promising of the new psycholeptic drugs." Meprobamate, he observed, was the best known because of attention in Hollywood. Overall, however, his summary of this drug's activity was quite positive.

Newsweek (1956a) reported that 5 percent of all Americans would take tranquilizers in a given 30-day period, and also that the consensus from a New York Academy of Sciences meeting was that "meprobamate, under proper medical supervision, is truly an *ideal tranquilizer*" [emphasis added]. Salutory results were reported in drivers, flyers, alcoholics, and heart attack and migraine victims. It was reported to be nonhabit forming. Earlier, *Science News Letter* (1956d) had reported good results with meprobamate "without undesirable side effects except for low blood pressure with large doses." *Newsweek* (1956c) reported that meprobamate helped heavy drinkers sober up.

Time (1956b), calling them "Don't-Give-A-Damn Pills," described Miltown as "the fastest selling pacifier for the frustrated and frenetic." A national shortage was described, which was most acute, according to this account, in Hollywood. The article was accompanied by a picture of a mugging "Miltown" Berle.

Coronet (1957) called them "Peace of Mind Pills" and although attention was given to side effects, this article dealing with chlorpromazine and reserpine mainly was generally positive: "The drugs do not by themselves cure sick minds; they benefit the patient by allowing him the peace of mind—the tranquility—in which to establish a more realistic outlook. They can be withdrawn when this has been accomplished." A brief report in *Science Digest* (1956), however, quoted concerns of one physician that some "mental" drugs might affect automobile driving.

Newsweek (1956c) gave some history of the tranquilizing drugs, noted the growing number of jokes about Miltown, and called them "happiness pills" and "emotional aspirin." Apparent shortages in drug store supplies were again noted, and some caution in use was suggested.

Time (1956a) gave a rundown on the status of "Pills for the Mind" then available. Compared with chlorpromazine and reserpine, meprobamate was reported to be effective in a smaller percentage of hospitalized patients, but to be the most popular with "millions of walkie talkie neurotics." *Look*, in July 1956, revealed "The Unhappy Facts About 'Happy Pills'." Little distinction was made between the major and minor versions, as the problem of diagnosis, the side effects, and paradoxical reactions were detailed. On balance, the article left the impression of overuse in the face of incomplete knowledge of how the drugs work (Berg 1956).

Also in September, *Christian Century* (1956), in an editorial on reserpine headlined "Happiness Pills Are No Answer," provided an interesting mixture of similies:

> Happiness pills and elixirs continue to be sought by those who want the satisfaction of a good life without a life that is good. Instead of grappling with the causes of unhappiness they seek merely to remove the symptoms. The same can be said of those pollyana forms of religious and political thought ranging from "positive thinking" to political piety, which are often allied to each other.

Life, in an article titled "The Search Has Only Started," described psychiatry as being in the same stage of development as medicine when "fever" was still considered a disease rather than a symptom of such specific conditions as pneumonia and typhoid. The discovery of bacteria made an enormous difference for medicine, but the "bacteria" of mental disorders had yet to be discovered (Hodgins 1956).

In general, this report gave the tranquilizers, just two years old, good marks, but already the question of how much tranquility in healthy in a society had begun to be raised. Nevertheless, there was considerable optimism. The head of the NIMH was quoted as saying: "I feel like Buck Rogers at this point." Indeed, the subhead for this article read, "In the next 10 years doctors may learn as much about the mind as in the past 2,000."

Science News Letter (1956b) reported on a study that found it safe to drive while taking meprobamate, and in a separate article stated that the drug was effective in relieving hangovers. The same issue quoted a professor of medical history as saying that tranquilizers would change medicine as much in the next 10 years as antibiotics had in the previous 15 years.

Business Week (1956) quoted the president of one major producer of the tranquilizers:

> The tranquilizer business is so terrific that retail prescription sales may top $25 million this year and may double in 1957. Such estimates promise to gilt-line the pocketbooks of producers, but a sobering fact can't be overlooked. The public is rushing to buy a panacea for tension and its handmaiden—anxiety—but many facts are still needed before medical experts can assess the public health and social consequences of their use.

Business Week continued: "A nation of tranquilizer addicts might well lose some of its intellectual drive, and some doctors rate this as No. 1 among the hazards involved in widespread use of the drugs."

In 1957, the American Medical Association (AMA) consumer publication, *Today's Health*, described the tranquilizers as "the peace of mind drugs" (Scott 1957). It described Equanil and Miltown as "younger cousins" of chlorpromazine and reserpine, no doubt adding to the belief that the drugs were all cut from the same cloth. Further misinformation may have resulted from the incorrect assertion that refills of meprobamate were prohibited by state law.

The same year, *New Republic* (1957) quoted a *New Yorker* cartoon: "Now remember," the wife admonishes her husband as he departs for the office, "You skip your tranquilizer. Watch for him to take his. Then hit him for a raise." The article still lumped the major and minor tranquilizers together in a generally negative article entitled "Domestic Tranquility."

Reader's Digest had already condensed a *Women's Day* article entitled "Happiness Doesn't Come in Pills," in which it was charged that Americans were spending $100 million to run away from normalcy—what the author called "Problems of Living." That same author, Arthur Gordon (1957), expressed views that were to be repeated in different forms by laypersons and medical personnel for the next quarter-century:

- Anxiety is normal and a pill will not make its specific cause disappear.
- Americans "haven't been trained to face trouble."
- Anxiety is a necessary part of a human warning system, and a sign of life.
- Happiness doesn't come in pills.

Science News Letter (1957c) reported on a veterinarian who had pet owners give their pets meprobamate before bringing them to his office. In February (Robinson 1957), the same magazine led with the statement, "Using tranquilizers can lull doctors, patients and parents into a false sense of security." The article summarized a paper on tranquilizer use in children.

Time (1957b), searching for new terms, found "Happiness by Prescription" and quoted a Beverly Hills psychiatrist: "I wish the Government would subsidize slot machines for tranquilizers on every corner."

Time was expressing concern about tranquilizer use in the article. One general practitioner was quoted as saying that tranquilizers "are not a substitute for compassion, understanding, patience, and attentive ear...."

These drugs should not be prescribed as an alternative for psychiatric therapies." And there was still confusion between the major and minor tranquilizers, with chlorpromazine and meprobamate mentioned in the same article with little distinction made between the two. *Time* did note, however, that refill restrictions were already being applied to the latter in several states.

The next month, *Science News Letter* issued a favorable report on the major tranquilizers (Robinson 1957) but paraphrased a research study on meprobamate to human terms from a study on rats: "This would mean that you might still feel scared when you see a car speeding toward you [after taking a tranquilizer], but the fear would not make you run."

American Mercury, in an interesting historical approach, argued that "it has become possible of men to annul . . . frustration artificially, enjoy a simulated happiness without paying the heretofore prevailing price, it is not reasonable to assume that the pace will slacken, cease to move, and begin to slip backwards?" (Raley 1957). The same month, *Harper's* presented an extensive analysis of the tranquilizers, which considered them all a part of a group even though "their pharmacological actions vary somewhat" (Stevenson 1957). The author, a physician, saw the role of tranquilizers at that time as preparing the patient for recovery. In a tidy simile, he noted, "Tranquilizers help the psychiatrist as morphine helps the orthopedist by dulling the pain while he sets the fracture." Even at this early point, he may have identified the two principal determinants of the future success of the tranquilizers:

> A physician cannot give someone a pill without also communicating at least two messages to him. First, "I am interested in you and I will take care of you." Secondly, it implies, "If you take this medicine you will become better." Thus, the physician offers the patient interest and hope. (Stevenson 1957)

Similar to other comments about the fashion cycle for drugs, Stevenson quoted the nineteenth-century physician Trudeau in advice to young physicians, "Make haste to use new drugs while they are still effective." (This very literate and incisive article both preceded and anticipated in content scores that were to follow it.)

Science Digest (1957) noted that "You Can Be Too Tranquil," and quoted research reports suggesting that meprobamate may reduce fears needed to escape danger, e.g., auto collision. The next month, however, *Farm Journal* (1957) reported that chlorpromazine and reserpine helped hens lay better, thus, perhaps, putting a touch of whimsy back into the picture.

When *Science Digest*, in November 1957, reported that the army had grounded all pilots using tranquilizers, they also reported tests at the University of Michigan on the effects of meprobamate on driving. Noting that the tests gave a "clean bill of health," the article urged continued study of the "new influence on the American scene" (Meyer 1957).

Farm Journal (1958b) continued its aggressive coverage of the tranquilizers. Feeding "tiny" amounts of tranquilizers to pigs, according to one report, resulted in 13 percent faster weight gain on 8 percent less feed. Further, the use of drugs was suggested prior to shipping and slaughter. As one feeder put it: "It surely took all the snort out of them."

For humans, however, *Consumer Reports* (1958) included a brief quotation from Surgeon General L. E. Burney, warning that "problems of daily living" [note the phrase] cannot be solved "with a pill," and the next month *Time* (1958c), under the headline "Drugged Failure?", was asking if the new psychiatric drugs were only "harbingers of a parade of drugs to cure and alter mental problems and capacities." *Time* reported that the Japanese were "wild for 'tranki'" (tranquilizers, mainly meprobamate). In Japan, no prescription was required and the advertising apparently rivaled U.S. promotion of Alka Seltzer. Billboards and newspaper ads were used. (Ironically, the Japanese manufacturers were concentrated in Osaka, around a shrine of Yakusoshin, an ancient god of drugs.)

Science News Letter, in March 1958, reported on a prison study, the results of which showed meprobamate not to be habit forming, but *Newsweek* (1958), the same month, noted an announcement of the beginning of hearings by Congressman Blatnik into advertising (excessive) of prescription tranquilizers (unnamed).

Business Week (1958) "covered" the AMA convention and suggested considerable behind-the-scenes fighting over the efficacy and safety of the tranquilizers. The same article contained photos of Salvador Dali's exhibit on "man's release from anxiety." The exhibit was sponsored by Wallace Laboratories and consisted of a 60-foot "chrysalid" or "butterfly cocoon."

The autumn of 1958 brought two disparate articles. *America* quoted Pope Pius XII as urging ethical sensitivity in the use of tranquilizers, whereas *Farm Journal* (1958a) passed along the news that Pfizer had received permission to add Tran-Q (hydroxyzine) to beef feed as a growth booster. A combination expected to follow was hydroxyzine, terramycin, and stilbesterol.

The *Farm Journal* article was followed by a 1959 *Coronet* article (Robinson 1959) reported on "Happy Pills for Animals" and quoting one veterinarian as saying; "Since [the tranquilizers] introduction, animals have entered an era of freedom from pain and suffering that was unthinkable just three years ago." Reports from zoos and pig and turkey farms seemed to confirm a new age of tranquility for the animals (Robinson 1959).

Science Digest (1959) quoted a *Journal of the American Medical Association* article that said that tranquilization is harmful to emotional health because of "the 'malignant tendency' forcing us to believe that no one should ever be afraid or so moved about his position in life that he does something about it."

THE 1960S

By 1960, the Kefauver hearings were in full sway. *Science News Letter* (1960b) quoted the Kefauver proceedings that Americans spend $280 million annually on tranquilizers. *Newsweek* (1960), also covering the hearings, suggested that huge profits were being made, and *Time* (1960d) described the hearings as "Trouble in Miltown" because of their focus on the pricing of Miltown and its competitor Equanil. *Business Week* (1960) added reports of price fixing by Wallace and American Home Products.

Back on the medical scene, *Science News Letter* (1960a) quoted one physician as calling the prescribing of tranquilizers a "doctor disease." He claimed that four types of physicians were prone to prescribe such drugs: (1) those who have trouble communicating; (2) those who have no alternative to offer; (3) those who want to please; and (4) those who cannot stand anxiety themselves.

Time (1960c), in one of the first reports of a new drug and a new era, described the taming of a lynx in the San Diego Zoo with Librium: "Librium comes close to producing pure relief from strain without drowsiness or dulling of mental processes." The same month, however, *Science News Letter* summarized a Washington conference on psychotropic drugs in a negative article, suggesting that general practitioners may be "doling out the calming pills to relieve their own anxieties which develop when they do not know what to do for a patient" (Davis 1960).

A lengthy article in *American Mercury*, in April 1960, dealt with mind control. Expressing a grave concern about research on human behavior, the author attributed to Aldous Huxley the theoretical view that "only neurotics and psychotics should receive tranquilizers, rather than the millions of sane people who do take them." He called behavioral science a "euphemism for mind and body control," and stated outright that "sodium fluoride added to drinking water is another method of mind control" (Benedict 1960).

That same month, the *Nation* published a report on the then ongoing Kefauver hearings. Written by a historian, the article criticized the industry as a whole but finished with the observation: "Beyond Huxley, I have found no study by an anthropologist, sociologist, psychologist, psychiatrist, philosopher, or any combination of these, on the impact of the tranquilizers on man and his culture" (Cowen 1960).

In May, Librium ("a new 'peace of mind'" drug) turned up again in *Time*, and this time it was not such a glowing report. It contained case studies of bizarre behavior in patients of one psychiatrist who admitted giving doses of 75 milligrams per day. A group of psychiatrists who reviewed the cases, however, "agree[d] that with the right dosage and for the right type of patient, Librium is a useful drug" (*Time* 1960a).

American Mercury (1960) presented a series of quotations under the title, "To Tranquilize or Not to Tranquilize." All were negative, but *Today's Health*, in November, told "The Story of Tranquilizers" in a very positive article.

In 1962, six years after its first description of the tranquilizers, *Changing Times* took another look. By this time, the magazine stated that "most psychiatrists agree [that] the psychic drugs have been at best only modestly successful and very often failures, for run-of-the-mill anxiety and depression." A continuing theme was the symptomatic, not curative, results.

Listed among the minor tranquilizers then extant were Miltown/ Equanil, Ultran, Soma, Atarax, Suavitil, and Librium (the last incorrectly identified as being in the diphenylmethane family). Addiction and withdrawal were mentioned as possible bad effects.

Reader's Digest in July referred to the tranquilizers as "a Turkish bath in a tablet" in a generally cautionary article that mentioned only chlorpromazine (Hartley 1962). According to a report the next month in *Science Digest*, meprobamate and chlordiazepoxide had, in practice, been used principally in aiding the therapist in treating patients suffering from neuroses, stress disorders, and alcoholism. "In these conditions minor tranquilizers usually produce results as good as, but not convincingly better than conventional forms of treatment with psychotherapy and older, more inexpensive sedatives" (Hordern 1962).

Popular Science Monthly, in February 1963, described its article as "The Truth About Brain Drugs," and devoted it to an explanation of brain functioning (Steen 1963). In May, *Better Homes and Gardens*, in a generally cautionary article, suggested alternative nondrug therapy (Green 1963). (In an interesting juxtaposition, the page on which this article appeared was shared by an ad showing a young woman, arms thrust in the air, saying "Free" seven times. It was an ad for Tampax but could easily have been for Miltown.)

By October 1963, *Good Housekeeping* in its "Better Way" section was turning its attention to the nonprescription tranquilizers, noting that the "use of [prescription tranquilizers] is effectively controlled because prescriptions *are* required to buy them." The consensus was that over-the-counter drugs were both ineffective and dangerous. Walter Modell, an eminent pharmacologist, was quoted as believing that "no drug for sleep or to reduce tension should be sold without a physician's prescription."

The next year, *Newsweek* (1964b) used the term "tranquilizer decade" and pointed out (inaccurately) that "in any reputable pharmacy, some 75 different compounds bearing more than 100 trade names in every conceivable color are visible." They quoted a Baylor psychiatrist, T. H. Greiner: "The milder tranquilizers are used sort of like vitamins." After some good words about the effects on psychotic patients, the side effects and social problems were highlighted in what use, on balance, a negative article.

In its April 30, 1965, issue, *Time* reported the deletion of meprobamate from the *U.S. Pharmacopeia*. Among reasons cited were a growing disillusionment among physicians concerning its effects as well as reports of addiction and withdrawal symptoms. Interestingly, the article was titled "Let Down for Miltown," although Equanil was also affected. (Perhaps rhyming was a problem, although "Bitter Pill for Equanil" does come to mind.)

The next year, *Science News* (July 9, 1966a) reported on efforts to determine which parts of the brain are affected by meprobamate. The results were inconclusive, though similarities to the other substances reportedly led to calling meprobamate "weak barbiturate" or "weak alcohol." It was also reported that evidence had been cited showing meprobamate to be addictive. Earlier, *Science News* (1966b) had reported on a symposium on "mind-acting" drugs. Among the items—the suggestion that meprobamate works on higher intellectual functions, whereas chlorpromazine affects arousal and attention.

In 1967, *Consumer Reports* did one of its patented reviews, this time on the psychoactive drugs. Beginning with quotations from medical advertising for the drugs, they decried the use of uncontrolled trials in evaluating them and implied that when good controls are established, the minor tranquilizers fare little better than do placebos. The next year, however, a *Good Housekeeping* article (1968) entitled "How Can Drugs Affect Mental Health?" used the term "minor tranquilizers," and concluded that (1) The drugs are relatively safe in small doses; (2) Effectiveness is still in question; (3) Some medical authorities believe they are overprescribed; and (4) They can be addictive. In 1969, *Transaction* reported on Parry's paper [from *Public Health Reports* (1968)]. According to Parry, as reported here, the "psychotropes" (sedataives, tranquilizers, and pep pills) are used as alternatives to alcohol.

THE 1970S

The 1970s opened on a negative note, as *Transaction* published a lengthy criticism entitled "Pharmaceuticals: Valley of the Lies," which leveled various familiar economic and marketing charges at the drug industry but which did not mention the tranquilizers (Gewirtz and Graham 1970). *Consumer Reports* (1971b) followed this with a list of "Medicines You May Want to Avoid." The list included tranquilizer-hormone combinations such as PMB-200/400 and Milprem-200/400.

The next month, *Consumer Reports* (1971a) in an article, "More Drugs to Think Twice About," simply listed the drugs identified by the FDA as "possibly effective," i.e., those for which little evidence of effectiveness had been found. Among the scores of drugs on the list were Listica, Trepidone, Darvo-Tran, Ultran, Suavitil, Meratran, Quiactin, Deprol, and Nardil.

McCall's reviewed some of the criticism of drug advertising featuring women as models as well as the proportionately higher rates of tranquilizer prescribing for female patients (Berg 1971).

Nothing of note appeared in 1972, but in 1973 (the year in which many observers report that the decline in use of minor tranquilizers began), *Science News* published an article entitled "Catch 22 of Psychopharmacology." The material came from Blackwell's articles that had appeared in the *Journal of the American Medical Association* and in the *Archives of General Psychiatry*. In these, Blackwell had suggested that prescribing by physicians, not patient demand, was the major factor in overuse of the drugs.

Today's Health, the AMA consumer magazine, in 1974 provided a "comprehensive evaluation of the *over-the-counter* tranquilizers" (italics mine). The evaluation—they are no good (Norman 1974). *Good Housekeeping* (1974) described "When Tranquilizers Are Dangerous" and quoted "authorities" as saying the drugs "are safe when used as directed by a doctor." They then provided guidelines for safe use. One interesting note: *Good Housekeeping* stated in concluding the article that it had declined advertising of over-the-counter calming agents "because of unresolved questions as to their effectiveness and the possible hazards of unsupervised use."

John Pekkanen, well known for his book *The American Connection*, wrote in the *New Republic* in 1975 that Librium and Valium had "just fallen under government regulation" (of course, he meant Drug Enforcement Agency (DEA) control, FDA having long regulated all drugs). This article told that story. Among other items included in this very negative article were references to the 1963 article in *Life* in which Librium was shown to be effective in tranquilizing a lynx. "Forevermore," Pekkanen said, "Librium would be known as the drug that tamed wildcats." He also made the incredible statement that "only about two percent of the sales income of these drugs goes to manufacture and distribution. The remaining 98 percent is for promotion and profit" (Pekkanen 1975).

In June 1975, *Science News* reported on the "scheduling" of Valium and Librium and quoted a GAO (Government Accounting Office) study in Veterans Administration hospitals. The report noted that efficacy was not in question, but rather the patterns of use. *Vogue* (1975) contributed its own warnings in "Danger Ahead! Valium—The Pill You Love Can Turn on You." The article began with a quotation from psychiatrist Marie Nyswander concerning the danger of Valium: "A far worse addiction than heroin, morphine, or meperidine [Demerol]." She said, "If you are taking 200 to 300 milligrams of this drug [daily], you probably can't stop." Indeed! But she didn't mention that this is 20–30 tablets of the highest dose of Valium—clearly abusive and (one hopes) a regimen no physician would prescribe.

Given the opportunity to be strident, Deborah Larned presented a very well-balanced picture of Valium in a 1975 issue of *Ms.* Oddly, in this magazine frankly aimed at women, Larned never mentioned the high rate of use among women compared with use by men. She did suggest the need for a patient package insert similar to that provided with oral contraceptives. "Perhaps most important," she said, "users should be informed that Valium does not 'cure' anxiety and, advertising messages aside, has never been shown to be an effective 'treatment' for such things as reluctance to do housework" (Larned 1975).

Late in 1975, the president of Hoffmann-La Roche was quoted: "Our principle is that we do not enter a field unless we can play first violin." The article, "The Selling of Valium," was critical of advertising of the drug, which appealed "to needs and biases" of the physician. This time the male-to-female use ratio was noted. "It's no wonder," the article concluded, "that the majority of tranquilizer users in this country are women" (*Ms.* 1975).

The *New York Times Magazine* called the widespread use of the best seller "Valiumania." They noted the derivation of the name—from the Latin for "to be strong and well"—but pointed out that "some critics go so far as to say that it is doing more harm than good" (Cant 1976). The article quoted Marie Nyswander, again, as asserting that Valium is "the most addictive drug in common legal use," but noted that she stands virtually alone in that view. Among the other concerns discussed were teratogenicity, impotence, and overpromotion. The history of the mental drugs was again reviewed, as was Sternbach's "discovery" of the Librium gathering dust on a shelf. The article concluded;

If Valium is a major reliance in what moralists and some sociologists complain is a hedonistic, sybarytic culture, losing its git-up'n'-go drive and seeking nirvana in a little bottle of tablets, its use is a symptom rather than a cause of this condition. Properly used by the medical profession, it has only medicinal properties. A drug has no moral or immoral qualities. These are the monopoly of the user or abuser.

In April, *Vogue* interviewed Dr. Frank Berger (the "father of Miltown") and received, not surprisingly, a generally favorable view of the drugs (McClean 1976). The next month, in *McCall's* (1976), physician William Nolan provided medical guidelines for the use of minor tranquilizers in a genrally well-balanced article.

Ladies Home Journal (1976) published "Women and Tranquilizers," which covered some of the basic material on these drugs. The article suggested that greater use by women occurred because they do not have the outlet for tension of going into a bar for a drink. The article also explored the importance of role conflict: "[Valium use] simply can't be separated from the position of women in today's society." An unfortunate inclusion was a "Glossary of Tranquilizers" that included major and minor tranquilizers, antidepressants, and Ritalin.

Time, in the only article covering this issue in 1977, provided a brief research report warning against use of alcohol and tranquilizers at the same time. The next year, Annabel Hecht, an FDA staff writer, authored "Tranquilizers: Use, Abuse, and Dependency" for the official government publication *FDA Consumer*. Strongly negative in tone, the article noted the high frequency with which Valium was associated wih drug abuse and suicide attempts in women. Hecht is one of the few writers who compared female use of Valium with the use of opium: "Strinkingly similar patterns in prescription drug use and abuse were reported 10 years ago. Great grandma, too, was a drug abuser, but her chemical 'crutch' was opium" (Hecht 1978).

Hecht explored familiar ground in seeking explanations for the high rate of tranquilizer use and called Valium "Executive Excedrin." Her article ended with a foreshadowing of the diazepam patient package insert.

The Kennedy hearings on the benzodiazepines were underway in the fall of 1979, and *Time* (1979a) covered the story in an article entitled "Tranquil Tales." They, along with the television networks, quoted one drug-abusing doctor describing his wait for Valium samples: "Where other doctors read their mail, I ate mine."

Also quoted was physician Joseph Pursch, who ranked tranquilizer abuse second to alcoholism as the nation's major health problem. Roche's position that addiction incidence was low was noted, as was a 22 percent drop in the use of tranquilizers over the previous six years. It is notable that Pursch's comment that the pills "don't solve anything" was described by *Time* as a "familiar message."

Newsweek, in November of that year, published a multipage feature on drugs and psychiatry. Much of the article was used to describe the history of the subject and to attempt a scientific explanation of how some of the drugs function. Valium was cited as "unquestionabl[y] ... [having] a useful place," but it was noted that it may be prescribed too freely and also inappropriately (i.e., to depressed patients) by family physicians. The ultimate thrust of the article was the considerable growth in the understanding of brain chemistry, with the potential of major breakthroughs in the near future.

THE 1980S BEGIN

In 1980, just two years after the Hecht article, *FDA Consumer* published "Overcoping With Valium" (Anon., 1980b). The anonymous article was very negative, citing the suspicion that Valium, taken alone, caused some deaths. (The 1978 Hecht article had stated that "no deaths have been attributed to use of Valium alone.") Again, the report referred to plans for patient package inserts as well as proposed changes in labeling. Addictive problems and "overpromotion" were also highlighted.

In July, *Time* (1980b) published "Yellow Light for Tranquilizers"—in *Time*-ese, "Bottled Well Being," "A Placebo for Our Overmedicated Society." It was a news report of FDA labeling changes to include that "anxiety and tension associated with stress of everyday life usually does not require treatment with an [antianxiety] drug." The article also quoted Sidney Wolfe's suggestion of no refills and criticism of a Cornell continuing education program as a subtle promotional effort for Roche products. Earlier (1980c), *Time*, in an article entitled "Psychoprofits," had discussed financial problems with Valium. The report implied that Valium was a financial cause of concern for Roche, but never explained why. It concluded with a list of new drugs in research.

In June 1980, *Cosmopolitan*, in a broad view of several psychotropic drugs and drug classes, singled out Valium and noted that "tranquilizer popping may be largely unwarranted, since anxiety often subsides by itself or in response to reassurance." Addictive potential and overprescribing were also mentioned (Tucker 1980).

DISCUSSION

During the period 1955–80, in which these magazines were surveyed, a total of 114 articles were found that dealt in some way with tranquilizers,

TABLE 5.2. Tranquilizer Articles in Lay Periodicals by Year and Content

| Year | Number of Articles | | |
	Favorable	Unfavorable	Balanced or Neutral
1955	2	—	2
1956	14	7	—
1957	5	7	3
1958	5	3	5
1959	2	6	—
1960	2	6	1
1961	—	—	—
1962	1	2	—
1963	1	2	2
1964	1	3	1
1965	—	1	—
1966	—	1	—
1967	—	1	—
1968	—	1	—
1969	—	1	—
1970	—	1	—
1971	—	3	—
1972	—	—	—
1973	—	1	—
1974	1	1	—
1975	—	4	1
1976	1	1	3
1977	—	1	—
1978	—	1	—
1979	—	1	1
1980	—	4	—
Total	35	59	20

in most cases the minor tranquilizers. Table 5.2 contains a breakdown of the articles by year of publication and according to an admittedly rough and subjective classification scheme. In raw numbers of articles, two conclusions suggest themselves. First, the large majority of articles (more than 50 percent) appeared in the first five years of the minor tranquilizer era. Second, although favorable accounts predominated in the first few years, the balance quickly shifted to those with a negative view.

It should be noted that the figures in Table 5.2 have only limited utility. They do not take into account either the length and persuasiveness of the articles or the circulation of the magazines. Surely an article in *Time* could be expected to have a greater impact than one in *Science News Letter*, at least in terms of readership. As we noted earlier, the media surveyed represent only a part of messages received by the public since meprobamate first opened the door to the minor tranquilizer era. Perhaps the ultimate in media exposure occurred when Valium was given the "Sixty Minutes" treatment in 1980. Using a tactic for which the program would later be criticized, Mike Wallace, on the air, told Roche President Robert Clark at the beginning of the program that its female producer had succeeded in obtaining Valium from three different Denver physicians simply by telling them she had left her bottle at home.

The questioning was tough. ("Why do you push Valium so hard, Mr. Clark?") It was critical of Valium advertising as being akin to a soap opera. When Roche Director or Professional Services Bruce Medd described long-term use in children with cerebral palsy, Wallace admonished, "Forget cerebral palsy children."

The topics ranged from addiction to failure to warn of side effects, interaction with methadone, and "scheduling" of the drug, with such abrupt changes of subject as the following somewhat incongruous question: Wallace—"Have you ever heard of a poison center out in Denver?" And another: "Why does Hoffmann-La Roche stock, tell me, sell at $36,000 a share?" In yet another statement, Wallace referred to "lots of friendly pharmacists, who charge a little more for their Valium without prescription."

Writing in *TV Guide*, physician Michael Halberstam (1980) took strong exception to the "60 Minutes" segment on Valium. "Wallace," wrote Halberstam,

> had scented a great scandal in the Nation's use of diazepam, but apparently, no scandal had been forthcoming. Undaunted, CBS presented a textbook example of how to slant a feature story. After an initial disclaimer from a physician who pointed out that Valium is a helpful and valuable drug, the program proceeded to show nothing but abuse.

Among Halberstam's criticisms was the failure to show some of the drug's positive uses—jobs saved, family relationships maintained. According to him, "The aura of scandal had to be preserved, though its substance was clearly lacking."

It would seem to require no documentation to assert that Valium is the best-known prescription drug name in the country today. The same thing might have been said of Miltown a quarter-century ago. Certainly the lay periodicals had a role in popularizing these drugs, but it seems equally certain, based on the review presented here, that the press contributed as well to a healthy skepticism of both the medical and social roles of the minor tranquilizers and probably played a part in their decline.

6

TELLING THE DOCTOR

"Wery good thing is weal pie, when you
know the lady as made it and is quite
certain it ain't kittens."

Charles Dickens
Pickwick Papers

The minor tranquilizers were not a totally new concept—physicians
had long used barbiturates and other substances to calm their patients.
Nevertheless, the products historically used had been basically sedatives.
Meprobamate and later the benzodiazepines were different in their effects
and their intent. Somehow, as is the case with any new type of therapy, the
prescribing physician had to be told both of the existence of these new
drugs and how to use them.

There are a number of models of information flow to physicians (see
Miller 1974). The common denominator of such models is a two-part
information system: the professional (presumably accurate, objective, and
balanced) information system and the commercial, promotional process.
The minor tranquilizers were prominently included in both. Literally,
thousands of published papers and an equal assortment of commercial
messages were produced relevant to the minor tranquilizers. No practicing
physician will have read them all. Nor are they all reviewed here. Rather, an
attempt is made to provide a "flavor" of the information produced during
the first quarter-century of minor tranquilizer use.

THE PROFESSIONAL PRESS

Minor tranquilizers were introduced to the medical profession in the
April 30, 1955, issue of the *Journal of the American Medical Association*,

83

which contained back-to-back studies on meprobamate, the first by L. S. Selling and the second by J. C. Borrus. [Both were later to be roundly criticized by Laties and Weiss (1958), but following their appearance, each was widely quoted.] Selling's study on 187 patients concluded that "Miltown (this was before the days of using generic names) was of considerable value in anxiety and tension states." The most dramatic results were reported in cases of "tension headache." Of 27 cases, 23 reported recovery or sufficient improvement so that they were not bothered by it.

In a section titled "Comparison of Miltown with Phenobarbital and Placebos," Selling reported: "I have records of 19 of the patients treated with Miltown who had taken phenobarbital before coming to me for treatment. None of these patients preferred phenobarbital to Miltown." Sixteen patients who had been taking Miltown were given an identical placebo, and "all of them complained so much about the return of their symptoms that they had to be returned to Miltown therapy immediately." Selling's summary and conclusions are quoted directly.

> Miltown (2-methyl-2-n-propyl-1,3-propanediol dicarbamate) is a practical, safe, and clinically useful central nervous system depressant. It is not habit forming. Miltown is also useful in keeping alcoholics sober after withdrawal is completed, and it has much value in accomplishing withdrawal with a minimum of discomfort. Favorable results have also been obtained in neurogenic conditions of the skin, in abdominal discomfort, and in several kinds of headache. Miltown is an effective dormifacient and appears to have many advantages over the conventional sedatives except in psychotic patients. It relaxes the patient for natural sleep rather than forcing sleep. (Selling 1955)

Borrus tried the drug on 104 patients. He offered it to each with the statement, "I am going to give you this medication to see if it will help you." All but 32 reported some favorable effects and 24 patients "recovered." Borrus, too, noted the "absence of toxicity," both subjectively and objectively.

Three years later, Laties and Weiss (1958) conducted a comprehensive and critical review of the literature then available on the efficacy of meprobamate in the treatment of anxiety. They led off with the following quotation from one of the leading textbooks in pharmacology (Krantz and Carr 1958):

> There is perhaps no other drug introduced in recent years which has had such a broad spectrum of clinical application as has meprobamate. As a tranquilizer, without and autonomic component in its action, and fraught with a minimal [sic] of side effects, meprobamate has met a clinical need

in anxiety states and many organic diseases with a tension component. That it has met this clinical need is evidenced by the fact that it is the most frequently prescribed of all drugs today.

According to the authors, "Only a handful of the studies on meprobamate [met] these criteria"; and further, the two earliest and, at that time, most widely quoted papers (those of Borrus and Selling) were conducted in such a way as to render their conclusions meaningless.

Nearly 100 references, most of them to studies, were cited in this review, which reached the following conclusions:

1. There is no evidence that meprobamate can be distinguished from a placebo in treating anxiety in psychiatric outpatients.
2. There is no evidence that meprobamate is better than a placebo in treating anxiety in hospitalized and psychotic patients.
3. No good evidence is available demonstrating a difference between meprobamate and a placebo in the management of anxiety accompanying physical disorder.
4. There is evidence that meprobamate is better than a placebo in the treatment of outpatient alcoholics and some evidence for its efficacy in acute alcoholism, but no evidence that it is useful in managing chronic hospitalized abstinent alcoholics.
5. There is no good evidence that meprobamate is any better than a barbiturate in assuaging anxiety, but some evidence that it may not be as good.

Laties and Weiss were at pains to note that they did not conclude that meprobamate was not effective, only that the quality of research on the drug was so poor as to render a judgment impossible. Their concluding statement is a telling one, and touches, again, on the drug life cycle:

It should be evident that totally uncontrolled studies of the effects of a new drug, especially when the dependent variable is something as amorphous and elusive as anxiety, can be misleading. A striking testimonial to the validity of this statement is the way in which the popularity of new drugs runs through the well-documented cycle of panacea, poison, pedestrian remedy. (Laties and Weiss 1958)

Weatherall (1962) provided another of the early reviews of the tranquilizer drugs. He noted that the term itself, in wide usage, was less than ten years old. Quoting and accepting the phrase from a then current advertisement, "the successor to the 35 tranquilizers," he suggested "that either a considerable degree of accuracy is necessary in diagnosis to distinguish each of the conditions for which a different tranquilizer is necessary, or... more drugs have been put in the market than are therapeutically necessary." (The logic is appropriate; the business naiveté perhaps excusable.)

It is interesting that at this comparatively early date, Weatherall would observe that "the word 'tranquilizer' appears to add little but glamour to the older term 'sedative', and it is convenient to consider together all the drugs which can be used to make patients feel more comfortable, *complain less* [emphasis added], and perhaps work better." (Convenient perhaps, but certainly misleading.)

Weatherall described the role of the minor tranquilizers "for troubled or troublesome patients in general practice." Meprobamate, now several years old, was described from a review of other studies as efficacious "only when given in massive doses under hospital conditions" or when "associated with a suitable physician." He concluded that the barbiturates, based on the evidence then extant, were better than other drugs for anxious patients, if only because their dangers were more fully known.

Weatherall's final 1962 conclusion was as follows:

> The actual therapeutic effects genuinely ascribable to tranquilizers themselves are very small, though not completely negligible. In therapeutically effective doses they reduce intellectual and physical skills and are apt to cause various pathological effects. Practically nothing is known about their influence on behavior in ordinary social contexts such as at home, in a factory, or on the road.

This concern was to follow the tranquilizers. A report of the Committee on Public Health of the New York Academy of Medicine recommended that "there should be an educational campaign to change the present public worship of 'happiness' and 'tranquility.' This attitude on the part of many people produces an almost slavish dependence on psychotropic drugs" (Committee on Public Health 1964).

Hayman (1964), although primarily involved in a discussion of such hallucinogens as LSD, wondered also if the profusion of tranquilizers, euphoriants, and atoractics might not provide the prescriber with a "vicarious pleasure and relief of tension" through "a process of identification with the person receiving the drug." He further observed that "it appears likely that often pharmaceutical houses, doctors, and patients alike have all been influenced by the same basic need for 'tranquilization.'"

In late 1965, Davis would report that already there were 5,000 references on the tranquilizers. His review was cautious but favorable to chlordiazepoxide, while diazepam had not been the subject of enough double-blind studies to warrant comparison with its predecessor.

Generally speaking, the physician reading the medical literature of the

1960s must have suffered from some confusion. There was a residual pattern of lumping major and minor tranquilizers together in discussions of psychoactive drugs. Even in the 1970s, confusion remained. Klein (1975) was concerned about the use of neuroleptics (major tranquilizers) in anxiety in the mistaken belief that they were probably more effective than minor tranquilizers. He also coined the term "polypharmaceutical stew" to characterize the confusion.

The beginning of the 1970s seemed to mark the beginning of a period of (generally) serious and balanced review of the minor tranquilizers and their place in medical practice and the decline of testimonials. Attempts were made to assess the degree of morbidity that was amenable to treatment with these medications, the relative safety and efficacy of the various products, and, with the beginnings of the new science of pharmacokinetics, some of the real differences among a growing class of benzodiazepines.

Based on the statistics on their use, it appeared that this new class of drugs was remarkably effective. Yet this same widespread use was cause for expression of alarm. On the one hand, prescribing physicians had been provided an apparently effective therapeutic tool, and, on the other, they were told they used it too much and too often.

Hollister (1975) expressed this dilemma in the 1970s while listing the "Desiderata" for psychotherapeutic drugs:

> The ideal psychotherapeutic drug would (1) cure or alleviate the pathogenetic mechanisms of the symptom or disorder; (2) be rapidly effective; (3) benefit most or all patients for whom it is indicated; (4) be nonhabituating and lack potential for creating dependence; (5) not allow tolerance to develop; (6) have a low incidence of secondary side effects; (8) not be lethal in overdoses; (9) be adaptable both to inpatients and outpatients; and (10) not impair any cognitive, perceptual, or motor functions. No such drug exists, but to a fairly surprising degree many of the available drugs meet the majority of these desiderata. It has been both our blessing and our curse that we had effective drug therapy for emotional disorders before we had a science of behavioral pathology.

But was the therapy effective? In 1971 Greenblatt and Shader published a damning review of "the history of meprobamate, the tranquilizer whose widespread use has persisted for 15 years despite an increasing body of evidence that fails to demonstrate its efficacy." They noted the history of its development and marketing and emphasized the role of "enthusiastic optimism about the future of tranquilizers" resulting from the success of chlorpromazine and reserpine. Included in the influential forces cited was the "strange appeal" of the brand name, Miltown, as well as enthusiastic praise in the medical press for the drug that, at that time, had been claimed to provide symptomatic relief for some 31 conditions ranging from alcoholism to typhoid fever. Greenblatt and Shader quoted its developer, Berger, in his 1964 paper in the *Journal of Neuropsychiatry*: "The drug most needed is the one that would liberate our minds from their primitive and outdated ways. Meprobamate may be the first substance of this type." They backed up their disagreement with this evaluation by a harshly critical review of clinical studies on the drug, concluding that "most authors, in evaluating this body of literature have concluded that meprobamate, although pharmacologically distinct from the barbiturates, is no less toxic and no more effective in reducing anxiety than a barbiturate such as phenobarbital."

The authors, who went on to publish *Benzodiazepines in Clinical Practice* (1974a), ended their article with a clinical judgment and a social question:

> On the basis of presently available knowledge, the benzodiazepine group of anti-anxiety agents (chlordiazepoxide, diazepam, oxazepam) appears to be more consistently effective than either placebo, barbiturates or meprobamate. Yet their current usage is so vast that we question whether physicians have not joined the popular media and the pharmaceutical industry in promoting a world in which avoidance and "tuning out" become substitutes for other forms of mastery. (Greenblatt and Shader 1971)

Greenblatt and Shader were supported in their views by Katz, who, reviewing the antianxiety agents in 1972, discussed the success of meprobamate, which, he said, had never been fully explained.

> [It] may have been due to its effectiveness in relieving anxiety without producing excessive drowsiness, the desire of physicians for a non-barbiturate sedative, a well-organized efficient advertising campaign and the right time historically for the introduction of such an agent. These factors are listed in order of increasing importance.

The British, too, were concerned about the rationality of therapy. Derrick Dunlop, long a prominent figure in the British drug review process (head of the "Dunlop Committee"), presented U.K. data in 1971 from which, he stated, it was difficult "to avoid the reflection that the overworked medical profession in this country may be too ready to *pander* [emphasis added] to the 'wants' of the public rather than to prescribe only for what we conceive to be its 'needs'."

Dunlop suggested that the benzodiazepines had been prescribed so often that they must frequently be used as placebos. He also supplied the interesting observation that "the better the doctor the fewer he prescribes since a good doctor is a placebo to himself." He observed darkly that the British had other sources of psychic relief:

> Even in the days when the counters of pharmacists' shops were piled high with opium pills offering for a few pence oblivion for those pouring out of the dark satanic mills of the industrial revolution, British people preferred to seek their escape with Bacchus in Hogarthian gin palaces rather than with Morpheus the bringer of dreams.

The 1970s were characterized by frequent attacks on the use of the minor tranquilizers.

In a letter to the editor of the *New England Journal of Medicine*, Feinbloom (1971a) called for a debate on the use of tranquilizers in medical practice. He urged physicians not to sweep patients' problems with modern life and their own lack of time to deal effectively with those problems "into a pharmacologic closet," as he perceived drug ads in the journal indirectly to suggest.

DiMascio (1975) described the use of psychotropic drugs in the early 1970s as "legitimized drug abuse" consisting of overuse, underuse, and inappropriate use. He lay part of the blame on the fact that only a small percentage (20 percent in a survey he conducted) of medical schools offered formal courses in clinical psychopharmacology. This in turn meant that "the majority of physicians and psychiatrists fail to learn and utilize the latest research findings," often for many years. As DiMascio put it, "Thousands of articles have been written describing findings of research endeavors that lend themselves to application in pharmacotherapeutics. . . . The findings from such research only very slowly wend their way to the clinicians responsible for treatment."

Not everyone was down on the tranquilizers, however. Gerald Klerman (1971), describing himself as "an angry psychiatrist," defended the psychoactive drugs (primarily the major tranquilizers) during a major conference on their use. Here, and elsewhere, he called attention to "pharmacological Calvinism" (if a drug makes you feel good, it must be bad). As Klerman put it:

> Psychotherapeutically, the world is divided into the first class citizens, the saints who can achieve their cure or salvation by willpower, insight, psychoanalysis or by behavior modification, and the rest of the people, who are weak in their moral fiber and need a crutch, whether it is Thorazine, Miltown, or Compoz.

Sue Boe (1971), repesenting the Pharmaceutical Manufacturers Association at a major conference, discussed the philosophical issues associated with the use of "reality-altering" drugs. She raised the interesting question "of whether the physician should have the right to exercise his value judgments to the point of denying a patient a legal medication when his decision not to medicate is based on other than physiological considerations—not only in the case of psychotropics but, for example, in the supplying of oral contraceptives to an unmarried girl." When she stated that "the use of psychoactive drugs reflects [a] change in values, rather than causes it," she might have added that the pill was a result rather than a cause of the sexual revolution.

Physicians received reports of and guides to prescribing. Blackwell (1973a), in the *Journal of the American Medical Association*, published a review examining what drugs were actually being used and what types of illness they were prescribed to treat (in contrast to "which drugs should be used in partciular conditions"), and questioning whether "the drugs being used are appropriate and whether their extent of use is proper or excessive."

Blackwell graphically illustrated that the substantial growth in the rate of psychotropic drug use in the previous eight years had been due to the benzodiazepines, most of it attributable to diazepam (although a mislabeled graph made it appear to be due to chlordiazepoxide). Interesting, later publications would show that a decline in use began the following year.

Noting that profound semantic confusion and symptomatic overlap, Blackwell presented evidence suggesting that the names used to describe illnesses "are chosen to reflect the drugs available to treat them." The busy practitioner is confronted with serious problems of discrimination—first "the task of separating psyche from soma," then "attempting to tease apart depression from anxiety."

Following a systematic comparison of the choice of psychotropic drugs with the criteria for selecting them, Blackwell concluded that "the evidence supports what is happening everyday practice," i.e., use of the benzodiazepines. This must have been some comfort to the readers.

Davies (1973) outlined the treatment of depression and anxiety in almost cookbook fashion. Although describing "doctor involvement" with patients as more important than drugs, he described diazepam as "safe and effective" and recommended use of benzodiazepines because (1) They work better than placebo; (2) They do not "readily produce dependence"; and (3) They are not dangerous on overdosage.

Citing a study that showed a significant influence of physician attitude on drug response, Hollister (1973b) identified a moral for the practitioner: "If you are going to prescribe these drugs, at least try to work up some enthusiasm for them and try to communicate it to your patients." But he predicted that "unless physicians learn to use these drugs with restraint, political pressures stemming from the growing problem of drug abuse may lead to unwise constraints."

As though an echo, an anonymous editorial appearing in the *Lancet* in early 1973 expressed concern about the rate of use of the benzodiazepines. Noting a (then) annual rate of increase of 7 million prescriptions for diazepam, the author concluded that "at this rate the arrival of the millennium would coincide with the total tranquilization of America."

This theme was to be repeated in the *Lancet* by Tyrer (1974) who, though noting that "no other class of drugs has shown the versatility and relative safety of the benzodiazepines," also observed that "sales of benzodiazepines are increasing in geometrical rather than arithmetical progression, and if the trend continues total tranquilization of the population will soon be achieved."

Tyrer seemed to blame the number of prescriptions on the number of drugs available. He called on the pharmaceutical industry to develop "some safeguards to prevent unscrupulous firms from jumping on any bandwagon which happens to be commercially appealing." What those "safeguards" might be or how they might be accommodated in a free enterprise system was not disclosed.

In 1974, published papers seemed to focus on helping the prescriber do a better job.

Gardner (1974), in an editorial appearing alongside one of the Balter et al. studies (see Chapter 4), noted the results of that study that showed a certain caution in prescribing. He further observed that "this type of survey can provide needed feedback to the average physician as he is called upon to make prescribing decisions that have moral and social, as well as the more 'typically medical' consequences."

Hussey, in a 1974 letter to the editor of the *Journal of the American Medical Association*, cited studies as the basis for his recommendation that physicians who prescribe an antianxiety drug "would do well not to write the label rigidly, e.g., 'Take one tablet four times a day, before meals and at bedtime.' Rather the label should read, e.g., 'Take one tablet when necessary for nervousness (anxiety). Do not take more than four tablets a day.'"

Trethowan (1975) in a review of drug use statistics in England referred to "the relentless march of the psychotropic drug jaggernaut." Blackwell (1975b) attempted to characterize the size and nature of that juggernaut. In an article, "Minor Tranquilizers: Use, Misuse or Overuse?", questions and answers were provided as follows:

1. What drugs are being used? Minor tranquilizers, mainly Valium, one of the most widely used drugs in medicine.
2. What illnesses are being treated? Most of what primary care physicians see, they label "anxiety."

3. Are the appropriate drugs being used? Yes, since their criteria for drug selection fit the most widely used class, the benzodiazepines. The reason for the leadership of diazepam is unclear unless one ascribes it to marketing practices or "that physicians and their patients know something that the scientist as yet does not."
4. Is there misuse or overuse? The author cited two studies as evidence that there might be.
5. How can overuse be explained? Although no clear-cut answers emerge, Blackwell provided a scenario with some explanatory value:

> The busy practitioner who makes a habit of ending each interview with a prescription will, therefore, be gratified and rewarded by the response which many patients report. This sequence of events constitutes the Catch 22 of minor tranquilizer use; the more they are given, the more they seem to work, the more they are prescribed. Too often neither the patient nor the doctor pauses to examine the role of enquiry, discussion and reassurance.

In another paper the same year, Blackwell (1975a) pointed out the quandary of treatment in which "a drug that is given often as first choice quickly becomes a preferred drug" because of a combination of factors including placebo response and spontaneous remission. Conversely, the drug that is reserved for one reason or another is more likely to reach treatment-resistant patients and consequently be undervalued.

Lasagna (1977) reviewed the various diagnoses for which minor tranquilizers were often used and suggested that there is reason to believe not only in their anxiolytic effects, but also in the possibility that they "may ameliorate, in certain patients, somatic complaints affecting such systems as the cardiovascular or gastrointestinal," i.e., organ systems "known to be linked in important pathophysiological ways to the nervous system."

The same year Solow noted that antianxiety agents were used in patients with a primary diagnosis of mental disorder only 37 percent of the time. In general, they were used for anxiety associated with somatic complaints. Solow noted that the use of such drugs in somatic illness may be justified on "simple humanitarian grounds." Most therapeutic reviews, however, do not deal with the issue. "Psychosomatic pharmacology," according to Solow, seemed to be about 20 years behind the development of psychopharmacology. His discussion provides an interesting contrast to the criticisms (see Chapter 4) of use of the drugs in somatic conditions.

> Response to psychosocial stress may involve a number of vicious cycles. The experience of unpleasant affect in response to threat or loss may be accompanied by various physiological arousal patterns. These in turn

may produce somatic perceptions (e.g. palpitations, muscle spasms, tremor which can be interpreted as further threat) and thus intensify the unpleasant affects. Since psychosocial stress may increase an individual's susceptibility to physical illness as well as producing psychic distress, the ensuing somatic disorder may itself be perceived as threat or loss, and feed into the cycle noted above. The consequent physiological arousal may adversely affect the somatic disorder in yet another vicious cycle.

Do psychotropic drugs ameliorate psychic distress produced by somatic illness as effectively as they relieve distress produced by external events? Can they moderate the response to stress so as to interrupt the vicious cycles noted above, enhance the individual's capacity to cope with illness, and produce improvement not only in the psychological disorder, but in a coexisting somatic illness as well? Indeed, can psychotropic medication be used to prevent the susceptibility to somatic illness produced by a clustering of significant life events? (Solow 1975)

Following a review of the use of such drugs in pain and delirium and in ischemic heart, gastrointestinal, skin, liver and kidney, and chronic obstructive pulmonary disease, Solow implied that use of psychotropic drugs should be a part of the total therapeutic resources brought to bear on somatic problems.

Hesbacher et al. (1975a) offered the opinion that "undoubtedly, one of the reasons why psychotropic drugs are so extensively utilized by the family physicians is because patients and physicians alike regard them as palliatives." Their study of nearly 1,200 patients treated in 1970, however, led them to conclude that the patient was being well served. They stated:

Family physicians choose from a limited range of medications, generally utilizing those regarded as "most effective." They are similarly judicious in their choice of patients to treat in this manner. Only a portion of those patients designated as having emotional problems and prescribed pharmacotherapy. This combination of sufficiently symptomatic patients, treated with well regarded psychiatric agents, enhances patient changes of improving and should sustain the family physician as the "first line of defense against emotional illness."

Physicians, in effect, were being told they were doing all right. There were warnings, however. Greenblatt and Shader (1976), for example, were worried about the number of new drugs:

For reasons that can only be speculated upon, pharmaceutical companies often expend great efforts in attempts to market as "new" psychotropic drugs the active metabolic products (or precursors of such products) of drugs that are already in use. Such "offspring" drugs available for clinical use in the United States include desipramine, nortriptyline, and chlorazepate. It is doubtful that this practice benefits humanity, since the differences between the offspring drugs and the parent compound are usually academic. Clinicians should be suspicious of claims of uniqueness made about "new" drugs which are actually metabolites or precursors of metabolites of old drugs.

Giordano (1977) reviewed the pros and cons of the benzodiazepines in *Military Medicine*. He summarized their usefulness and limitations and urged rational pharmacology as the answer to the danger that governmental restrictions on their use might be "tightened to the point of ridiculousness." "We must," said Giordano, "resist the impulse to prescribe benzodiazepines simply because we can't think of anything else to do, because the patient comes in and says he wants it, or because we feel the need to 'do something.'"

Overall, the medical literature on the minor tranquilizers, apart from purely clinical studies, seemed to follow a pattern roughly consisting of:

1. A comparatively short period filled with mostly "glowing" reports.
2. Critical reviews calling for caution and careful study.
3. Reports of "overuse," viewed with alarm.
4. Suggestions that, in fact, the drugs may be used appropriately.
5. Guidelines for prescribing.

This pattern occurred in the professional, presumably objective literature. Change was also apparent in the world of advertising.

A FEW WORDS FROM OUR SPONSOR

It is very appealing to look to drug advertising to physicians as a possible cause of presumed overuse of psychotropic drugs, especially the minor tranquilizers. Indeed, such advertising must have an effect on such use or drug manufacturers would be unlikely to continue to expend funds for this purpose. Equally certain, however, is the fact that the role of advertising is an indeterminate part of a complex set of social, medical, behavioral, and economic factors that result in the psychotropic drug prescription. Attention to advertising in isolation may result in simplistic solutions.

Although social scientists and others have been at pains to analyze advertisements for psychotropic drugs, the physicians themselves have seldom been asked their opinions. When this has been done, some of the concerns about the effects of the ads seem a bit less serious.

As an example, Lion et al. (1979) included 50 psychiatrists in a study in which they were shown ads from two professional journals from which the names of the products had been deleted. Generally, few of the ads were found to be informative or viewed as esthetically appealing. In spite of the wide exposure of some of the ads, few of the drugs were identified.

There is a serious need for controlled, sophisticated study of the prescribing and drug-taking process as it relates to psychotropic drugs. Within this study, greater resources must be committed to serious study of prescription drug advertising. A comprehensive review of the literature on this subject provides little information on which to base sound policy.

The difficulty of reaching consensus on prescribing issues is empha-sized in a paper by psychiatrist Nathan Kline. Kline (1976) proposed active therapy for depression. He described depression as "the most undertreated of all major diseases," and further stated, "The discrepancy between the *availability* of treatment for depression and the actual *providing* of treatment is so great as to constitute a scandal."

It is interesting to note some of Kline's suggestions in the light of comments by others. In contrast to the view of Hemminki (1974b), for example, Kline encouraged the use of antidepressant medication in patients with dominantly somatic disorders that, Kline stated, "have an important enough psychiatric element at times to spell the difference between rehabilitation and nonfunctioning." In the face of considerable criticism of the overuse of antidepressants, Kline took the view that they are underused. "If there is the slightest doubt, and even at times on a presumptive basis, the patient should be given the benefit of a trial on antidepressants." In his paper, Kline encouraged greater use of the antidepressants by general practitioners, noting "the percentage of nonpsychiatrists attempting to treat depression is discouragingly small."

Private enterprise might do a better job of informing physicians than other information sources. It is unrealistic, however, to expect the advertiser to voluntarily provide physicians with all the information they need about all treatment alternatives to make the best possible choice. A judgment that advertising is effective, then, leads logically to a need for equally effective supplementary (and sometimes counter) measures to inform the physician fully to allow performance as the patient's agent. But what if advertising is not effective in influencing prescribing habits? Since, by definition, ineffectiveness means failure to influence to prescribe, this means that patients are paying, as a part of their prescription charge, for advertising activity that is worthless. Further, since physicians apparently spend some time with advertising, another patient outlay is the opportunity cost of physician time that might have been better spent in other activities, such as acquiring information from other sources.

From a social policy point of view, this poses a real dilemma.

Advertising that works almost certainly gives rise to the need for additional information expenditures. Advertising that does not work is almost certainly a social waste.

Effects on Prescribing

This section includes a summary of the evidence that drug advertising has the demonstrable direct or indirect effect of too much or otherwise inappropriate prescribing. It is likely that considerable evidence of the effect of advertising on prescribing volume exists in the files of drug manufacturers who have certainly conducted marketing research in this area. For obvious competitive reasons, the manufacturers do not publish such research. Consequently, this review must be limited to published work.

It will not be possible here to explore all of the issues related to the prescribing of psychotropic drugs, particularly the antianxiety agents. An attempt will be made, however, to provide ideas on the subject as provided by a number of other observers.

Feinbloom (1971b) told Senate investigators that

the unopposed influence of the drug companies with their lavishly financed marketing programs, the financial dependence of medical journals on drug advertising, and the whole question of how the doctor himself acquires new information are not examined in medical schools.

He went on to relate tranquilizer use in manpower problems:

It is the pressurized overworked general doctor, undertrained in managing emotional problems and ego-committed to "do something" who is most likely to regard tranquilizers as a welcome, simple, and seemingly inexpensive answer to difficulty-handled complaints.

Parish (1974) echoed this view: "Most doctors in practice today have had no formal training in learning to manage the burden of mental disorders and common anxieties which exist in the community."

In the face of inadequate training and urged to do something, the physician may find difficulty in achieving a sense of control of the situation. The need for such a sense of control does exist, but its effect on prescribing is not clear.

Lewis (1971) surveyed 65 Boston-area physicians in 1971 and found that 67 percent believed that other physicians prescribed too many tranquilizers. This was a small study in one area, but it allows two points for consideration. First, the findings are in conflict with the more systematic studies by Balter and associates and with the opinions of Kline that these drugs may be underused. Second, if the nondirective theory of questioning is at work here, the physician respondents may actually be reporting a belief that they themselves prescribe too many tranquilizers.

What is the role of advertising in this scenario?

Linn and Davis (1972) conducted a study among a random sample of physicians in the Los Angeles area to determine the importance of sources of information on new prescription drugs. Journal advertising was considered the most important source by 16 percent of the respondents. Those who indicated high acceptance of this source of information displayed relatively conservative attitudes on three indexes of attitudes toward psychotropic drug use.

Hemminki (1974b) studied prescribing patterns and personal characteristics of 47 Finnish general practitioners and determined that the more positive the attitude that the physician had toward the use of drugs for social problems and everyday stress, the more psychotropic drugs were prescribed (she used the work of Linn). No significance was found in the relationship between prescribing frequency and stated reliance on commercial sources of information.

Stimson (1975b) used anecdotal evidence to conclude that ads for psychotropic drugs define the problems of living in today's society as "treatable by doctors." He described these activities as follows:

> The solution to the problem is not to change those things in the person's life that cause the problems, but to change the person by correcting his or her brain chemistry. The consequence of such symptomatic treatment is that cure, in a medical sense of solving the problem once and for all, is not possible.

Without the intention of diminishing Stimson's argument, it is appropriate to point out that there are substantial numbers of researchers who believe that the mental symptoms are the result of changes in brain chemistry and that, at least in the future, chemical intervention is a very plausible solution.

Lennard and his colleagues (1971), in the compelling book *Mystification and Drug Misuse*, saw greater danger in the use of psychotropic drugs for everyday problems: "As more and more facets of ordinary human conduct, interactions, and conflicts are considered to be medical problems, physicians and, subsequently, patients become convinced that intervention through the medium of psychoactive drugs is desirable or required."

The development of the model, according to Lennard et al., is insidious: "Thus, when a physician prescribes a drug for the control or solution or both of personal problems of living, he does more than merely relieve the discomfort caused by the problem. He simultaneously communicates a model for an acceptable and useful way of dealing with personal and interpersonal problems."

Why is this allowed to occur? Feinbloom (1971a) says: "Doctors are overworked, as drug houses and patients know. Inexpensive technical solutions to human distress become irresistibly attractive." Feinbloom's letter to the editor generated considerable discussion. One of the readers asked and then answered a rhetorical question: "Why are people so easily victimized by irrational propaganda? The answer obviously is because they want to be convinced." The writer was referring to laypersons, but does the answer apply to physicians as well?

Latent Effects of Advertising

The issue of whether drug advertising is "educational" is a difficult one to resolve, and an old one. May (1961) gathered most of the surrounding facts into a published discussion nearly 25 years ago. He described the prescribing physician as "the funnel through which all ethical drug sales must pass." May's analysis is still applicable. The essence of it is that some advertising is specifically presented in the form of education, but that much advertising is educational in outcome; i.e., it teaches the physician to use the drug being promoted.

In the case of journal advertising, there is some evidence that this concern is justified. In several studies, physicians made no distinction between journal advertisements and their other content in citing medical journals as a major source of drug knowledge.

Another concern that has been expressed more frequently in recent years is the potential influence of the many journal advertisements on physician attitudes aside from the drugs themselves. One of the major criticisms is the possible sexist content of the advertisements.

Kunnes (1973) noted that advertisements for fixed-combination diet pills appear to fit the sexist description. Seidenberg (1971) pointed out that it is possible inordinately to use pictures of women as "sick" or disturbed and thereby "create the image of women as not only the weaker sex, but the sicker sex." Seidenberg (1974) in another paper referred to a ten-year personal study of psychotropic drug advertising in which he found that "at least two-thirds to three quarters of the ads show pictures of women to whom psychoactive drugs are to be given." Unfortunately, the data from this study were not presented.

Mosher (1976) described the portrayal of women in drug advertising as a "medical betrayal." She did not provide data to support her views, but did provide important medical principles that apply if her charges are valid. She noted: "Exaggerated stereotyping appears to minimize the need for complete medical diagnosis, encourages unwarranted drug prescribing, and reduces the status of the person, as a patient and as a consumer." Stimson (1975b) took a similar position when he reported in a nonquantified fashion on what appear to have been nonrandom, nonsystematic observations of British journal advertising for tranquilizers and for oral contraceptives. He concluded that the overall effect "reveals a consistently limited view of women."

Mant and Darroch (1975) used content analysis techniques to study nearly 500 drug advertisements that appeared over a seven-year period in two Australian medical journals. Comparisons were made between advertisements for "mood-modifying" and other categories of drugs, and significant differences were found. Greater use of pictures and of female models more often than males as well as sexual stereotypes characterized the advertisements for mood modifiers. Assessment of scientific appeal revealed no significant differences by drug types or sex of the patient.

Unfortunately, this study did not describe adequately the structure of the index of scientific appeal, did not specify whether the aggregate findings were controlled for advertisements that appeared more than once in the sample, and suffered from an apparent need to find sexual discrimination. The researchers, for example, referred to some of the models as "seductive," although how this evaluation was made is not clear.

Prather and Fidell (1975) concluded that women were shown more often than men in psychotropic drug advertisements than in advertisements for other types of drugs. In addition to stylistic differences, they found females to be portrayed as suffering "diffuse emotional symptoms," while men were suffering from "pressures from work or accompanying organic illness." The sample of ads was drawn from one state medical journal and three national journals, one issue randomly selected from each of five successive years.

Chapman (1979) found the deepest and most obscure messages in psychotropic drug ads. He argued that the ads "have a mythical dimension which parallels aspects of nature and functions of myth in traditional societies." Just as some "have argued that the Disney cartoons function as a vehicle for U. S. imperialist ideology," Chapman hoped "to demonstrate that the imagery of some medical advertising functions to legitimize and perpetuate certain views of doctoring, drugs, and patients that are commercially advantageous to the drug industry."

Using a simplified typology, Chapman found ads for psychotropic drugs which, he argued, promote such myths as

- Drug product as daily food (like cornflakes)
- "Mom" as sunshine
- Drug as part of afternoon tea
- Doctor as cyberneticist
- Doctor as Merlin

King (1980) conducted a content analysis of the 2,675 drug advertisements in the *American Journal of Psychiatry* for the period July 1959 to December 1975. Among her findings were the following:

1. When a person was shown alone in the ad, that person was female 57 percent of the time.
2. Repeated ads (as opposed to those appearing a single time) used women as the primary figure 41 percent of the time compared with 29 percent for men.
3. Women were shown as patients in 81 percent of ads for antidepressants, but men were in the majority (51 percent) of ads mentioning symptoms of anxiety and tension.
4. Subjective evaluation led to the conclusion that female patients were "put down" in the ads, and this conclusion was supported by a study of psychology students' perception of subjects shown in the ads.

In related studies, Smith and Griffin (1977) found that female models were only slightly more often associated with nonrational appeals in advertisements for psychotropic drugs than were males. Smith et al. (1977) also found that although obvious attempts had been made to render some advertisements "sexy," their degree of sexiness was comparatively low.

There is some evidence that sexual bias in the ads may be related to physician beliefs.

McRee et al. (1974) used a mail survey to 30 psychiatrists (23 responded) to study whether the respondents believed advertisements were sexually biased and the effects of any bias so identified. A majority (70 percent) of male respondents indicated that female models in advertisements were more likely to attract their attention. Several respondents felt that psychiatrists would be less affected by advertisements that implied that more women than men had symptoms of mental illness. Seventy-four percent believed that nonpsychiatrists might be led by the advertisements to believe that more women than men had symptoms of mental illness requiring medication.

Parish (1973) has raised the possibility (but presented no evidence) that drug advertising affects not only prescribing, but also diagnosis: "The pharmaceutical industry is responsible for the way its products are promoted and in so doing it often defines and re-defines indications for the use of drugs and so, not only has the industry influenced treatment, it has influenced diagnosis."

Whatever the ultimate conclusion on the effect of advertising on minor tranquilizer usage (if a conclusion is ever drawn), one inescapable observation is that the advertising has changed a great deal in the course of the first 25 years. The reasons for change include inter alia developing marketing techniques, regulation and unofficial pressure by the FDA (see Chapter 9), and changing approaches to anxiety itself. Some examples will serve to illustrate these changes.*

The early advertisements for meprobamate and its (almost) immediate competitors were especially important. They had the task not only of promoting the use of a specific brand-named product, but also of introducing the concept of the antianxiety agent.

Miltown and Equanil, of course, led the advertising parade. Miltown advertising focused on the effectiveness of the product (Figure 6.1), referring to its actions in "emotional and muscular tensions." Almost from the outset, the relationship between drug effects and "normal family life" was cited. Equanil advertisements, which were to be mentioned in Senate hearings for more subdued promotion, nevertheless suggested that anxiety was a "part of every illness" and suggested its use in hypochondriasis.

Meprobamate was followed promptly by a number of competing products, each with its own advertising message. The Atarax campaign was built around a "peace of mind" theme and was one of the early products with pediatric indications. Some 25 adult and 10 pediatric indications were listed for Atarax—"perhaps the safest ataraxic known."

The most ambitiously named product was Lilly's Ultran (the "ultimate tranquilizer"), which ultimately did not survive the marketplace. Ultran advertisements used three themes (Figure 6.2): quick action, chemical uniqueness, and unimpaired mental activity.

Early in the promotional history of the minor tranquilizers, the married housewife began to make her appearance. An advertisement for Pacatal noted that "only a short time ago, Doris never had time for the kids." Pacatal therapy "released this housewife from the grip of her neurosis," as the illustration in the ad clearly showed, even with the warning that it "should not be used for the minor worries of everyday life."

The introduction of Suavitil was picturefree. Instead, the manufacturer, Merck Sharp and Dohme, adopted a factual, all-print approach that, in appearance if not in content, anticipated the stringent FDA requirements that were to follow the 1962 Drug Amendments (see Chapter 9). The product was described as "essentially nontoxic" (Figure 6.3). The basic Suavitil ad was supported by numerous "reminder" ads that described the product as "often effective where other psychotropic agents fail." Suavitil was an "antiphobic" and "antiruminant."

All of the products were, of course, "new." Some were new in different

---

*Most of the examples presented here are from medical journals. Many other forms of promotion are used, of course, but they are difficult to illustrate.

1. Borrus, J. C.: J.A.M.A. 157:1? ....ril 30, ... 2. Sell..... S.: J.A.M.A. 157:1594, April 30, 1955. 3. Lemere, F.: ...thwest Med ..098, Oct. ..5. 4 Ban... B. and M.ocutti, C.: Lav. neuro-psichiat. 19:693, 1... 5. Selli.... ...: J. Clin.. Exper. Ps.... th. 17:7. arch 1956 6. Berglund. M., Blumenthal, B......lorch, H.:...... lak. 5.:3369, Dec... 1956. 7. ..el, H. A., Wood, J. A. and Dixon, H. H.:...w York Aca... c. 67:780, May 9. 1957. ..ollister..... .. Elkins, H., Hifer, E. G. and St. Pierr.....Ann. New York Acad. Sc. 67:789, May 9, 957. 9. Ga..... ..: Rass. med. 34:233, July-Aug. 957. 10... i, R. et al : J. Pediat. Praxis 20:27, ..g. 1957. .....g 1957. ...Anaes-thesist .07, Aug ... 12. Tucker, W. I.: Sout... M. J. 52:1111, Sept. 195.....5. Roland;... Attual. ostet. . 3(6).. 9, Nov.-Dec. 1957. 14. .....hacker, W.: Klin. Mona... 1. Augenh...2):224, 1958. .....hebianc... G. and Ceroni, T.: Oto-... ring. ital. 26(2):143, 1958. 16. ....o, G.: Minor.... 49:1914, 1958. 17. ..tuso, R. and ...tti, F.: A.. eurol. 3(1):36, J..... 1958. 18. .....Gazz. med. ital. ..49, Feb. 5.....astur, R. .: J. Indian M. Prof.... 13, Feb. 1958. ..., W.: Therap. G.....t 97:66, ... 1. Be..... ..: Lyon med. 19.... March 2, 1958. ...iglia, G.: Miner...... 10:218, M.. 15, 1958. .....lander, H. S.: ... Cardiol.]:345. ... 1958. 24. McClen...... Arch. Ped.... 75:101, M...... 25. Sprauer, V. J.. Internat. Rec. Med.. GP Clinics 171:..... 1958. 26. ....inson, R....... ..Robinson, H. M.,.. .: South. M. J. 51:.9, April 1958. 27..... S. and Pek.an, L.: Ne......ed. 58:1283, April 15, 1958. 28. Bouquerel, J., Naviau and .....ne: Ann. med. ....ycol. 11......ne 1958. 29. Reboul, F., Reboul. M. and Dorgeuille, C.: Maroc ...... 37:784, July 1958, 30. B..... ..: Lyon med. 200:825, Nov. 1958. 31. Larpnier, T. A.: Maryland M... 7:627, Nov. 1958. 32. Leuke.... Med. Klin. 53:2113, Dec. 1958.

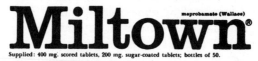
FIGURE 6.1

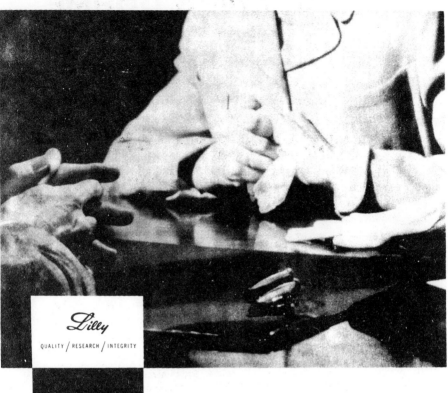

QUALITY / RESEARCH / INTEGRITY

release from anxiety

ULTRAN
(Phenaglycodol, Lilly)

mild, safe tranquilizer

anxiety quickly allayed

The patient with vague symptoms, nervous and distressed under the burden of unsolved problems, finds release from anxiety and restoration of emotional composure.

mental acuity not impaired

Exhaustive psychological testing shows that recommended dosage does not affect intellectual or motor abilities. 'Ultran' is the first drug for which this has been established by objective and standardized quantitative tests.

Dosage: Usually, 1 pulvule t.i.d.

Supplied: As attractive turquoise-and-white pulvules of 300 mg., in bottles of 100.

chemically unique

'Ultran' is a new chemical compound, one of a group of butanediols synthesized at the Lilly Research Laboratories. It is not a modification of any other therapeutic agent.

774030

ELI LILLY AND COMPANY • INDIANAPOLIS 6, INDIANA, U.S.A.

FIGURE 6.2

MERCK SHARP & DOHME
announces an important
new "psychotropic" agent

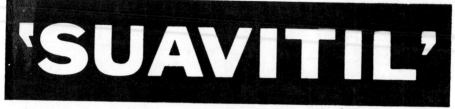

(BENACTYZINE HYDROCHLORIDE)

An entirely new approach to the medical problem of mild anxiety states, tension, depression and compulsion.

'SUAVITIL' relieves anxiety without producing depression or drowsiness ... assists patients to deal more constructively with the situations which produced such anxiety.

'SUAVITIL' differs fundamentally from any of the substances currently used in this field. 'SUAVITIL' has been reported to be, in many cases, the only agent indicated in the treatment of depression.

'SUAVITIL' causes no euphoria and leaves the quality of thinking virtually unchanged. It imposes no sedation and has no hypnotic effect, although it relieves sleeplessness by reducing repetitive thinking (futile rumination).

What it is

'SUAVITIL' (benactyzine hydrochloride) is a centrally acting psychotherapeutic agent with selective activity on various functions of the brain. It is believed to act essentially by inhibiting the transmission of nerve impulses between neurons.

'SUAVITIL' may best be described as an antiphobic, antiruminant, "mood normalizer". It has been extensively used in England and Den-

mark, and clinicians report that it effectively relieves tension, anxiety and depression in a majority of their psychoneurotic patients. Subjective benefits have been described by patients in the following terms: "I feel calm"; "It is a feeling of well-being"; "I feel soothed".[1]

What it does

'SUAVITIL' offers a new and specific type of neurochemical treatment for the patient who is disabled by anxiety, tension, depression, or obsessive-compulsive manifestations—whether the anxiety is founded in fact or whether it has become a neurotic state, out of proportion to environmental stimuli.

Absorption and tissue distribution

'SUAVITIL' is well absorbed and rapidly distributed in all tissues. However, except for CNS tissue it is rapidly metabolized out of all other tissues. Onset of effect is rapid, within 20 to 30 minutes.

FIGURE 6.3

ways. Softran featured a chewable tablet that "can be taken anywhere, anytime, no water needed." Quiactin ("for quieting" in case one overlooked the significance of the name) offered "wide awake tranquility" and demonstrated it with a photo of an elderly woman threading a needle.

As the number of products increased, attempts at product differentiation (beyond merely being "new") began. Tentone was a phenothiazine compound "for the lower and middle range of disorders" and demonstrated graphically its position between the other phenothiazines and the "mild ataractics." Trancopal was introduced as a "tranquilaxant," i.e., both a potent muscle relaxant and an effective tranquilizer. Ads showed patients engaged in physical activity apparently free from both low back pain and dysmenorrhea.

By 1959, Atarax, the "passport to tranquility" (Figure 6.4), was endorsed by the additional claims of being "antihistaminic, antiarrhythmic and antisecretory." At the same time, Vistaril (the same drug as Atarax, but marketed by another division of the same company) was being described as "more than a tranquilizer," although only the antihistaminic effect was

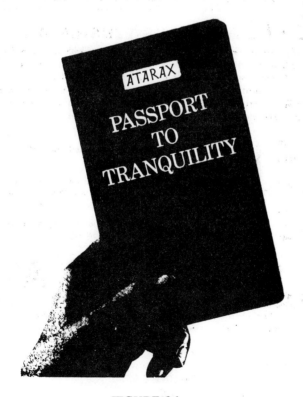

FIGURE 6.4

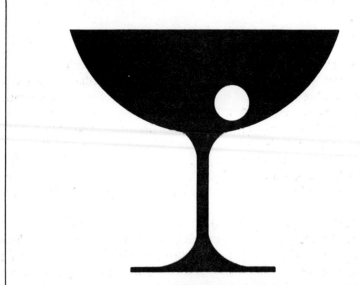

The Cocktail Glass- symbolizing tension / anxiety caused by men's inability to accept reality, and his occasional surrender to acute or chronic alcoholism.

LISTICA® ALLAYS TENSION/ANXIETY

LISTICA allays tension/anxiety...promotes eunoia*. During almost four years of clinical study involving patients with a wide range of conditions, Listica has proven 8·9% effective. Only 4% of patients have experienced even minor side effects, with the most frequent reaction being mild drowsiness during Listica therapy. Investigators have not reported any toxicity, contraindications, habituation, or cumulative effects or withdrawal symptoms.

LISTICA®
is recommended
for the relief of
anxiety and
tension
states
associated
with

- **Alcoholism**
- **Allergy**—Asthma, hayfever, rhinitis, sinusitis, dermatitis
- **Anxiety** and **Neurosis**
- **Bronchial Asthma** and **Bronchitis**
- **Cardiovascular Disease**—Angina, coronary disease, hypertension
- **Dermatology**—Neurodermatitis, herpes zoster, pruritus, urticaria
- **G.I.**—Peptic ulcers, ulcerative colitis, hemorrhoids, regional ileitis
- **Headache** due to tension
- **OB-GYN**—Menopausal, premenstrual tension, obstetrical anxiety
- **Surgery**—Pre- and postoperative anxiety
- **Trauma**

℞ **LISTICA**®

A NEW TENSITROPIC† ARMOUR PHARMACEUTICAL COMPANY • Kankakee, Ill.

Physicians who prefer generic names prescribe "Hydroxyphenamate, Armour"

*eunoia: A normal mental state (Stedman's Medical Dictionary).   †Favorably alters tension/anxiety

FIGURE 6.5

106

added to its psychotherapeutic potency. Dartal (perhaps because there was nothing new left to say) was promoted as "an outstanding tranquilizer for general use." Listica appeared to be an alternative to the cocktail (Figure 6.5).

By late 1960, a product was in the wings about to do mischief to these and the many other minor tranquilizers whose appeals were being presented to the practicing physician.

Moskowitz (1960) presented the marketing case history of the new product, Librium, in the trade journal *Drug and Cosmetic Industry*. He noted the growth of the tranquilizer market from 3 products in 1955 to 13 products in 1957 to 27 products (and $150 million) in 1959.

In the first three months on the market, Librium became the most prescribed tranquilizer.

Moskowitz presented data on early 1960 sales as shown in Table 6.1. His description of the Roche marketing campaign for Librium is interesting as well as being one of the few published case studies in the literature of prescription drug marketing. By his account, Librium advertising was assigned by Roche's William Gulick to the William Douglas McAdams Agency. Among the promotional efforts were the following:

- The Roche Record Report, a booklet left with physicians that contained long-playing records of physicians reporting Librium results
- Eight-page inserts in medical journals
- Forty separate mailings to physicians in the period March to July
- Only very limited use of samples

According to Moskowitz, Roche took as its marketing target all other tranquilizers and did so by means of a very confident but low-key message as quoted here:

At this time, Roche Laboratories introduces a new psychopharmacologic agent: Librium. In other words, another tranquilizer? Another tranquilizer, yes, in a manner of speaking. That is, insofar as it allays anxiety, tension and agitation, Librium could perhaps be called a tranquilizer (we see no point in coining a new, fanciful descriptive term). But Librium has several noteworthy properties that distinguish it from any "tranquilizer" you ever heard of or used . . . and it is very definitely *not* just another addition to an already lengthy list. Isn't that a rather familiar claim? Perhaps. In this message, however, we would like to transmit to you our own profound conviction that Librium *deserves* to be made available to the medical profession—despite (or possible because of) the existing compounds—and to let you share the enthusiasm of the many investigators (some of whom originally approached Librium with a certain

TABLE 6.1. New Prescriptions of Tranquilizers in 1960

	January	Percentage Change	March	Percentage Change	April	Percentage Change	June
Librium	—	—	60,000	+233	200,000	+60	320,000
Equanil	375,000	−20	300,000	—	300,000	−8	275,000
Compazine	300,000	−3	290,000	−10	260,000	−31	180,000
Thorazine	150,000	—	150,000	−13	130,000	−23	100,000
Miltown	140,000	−11	125,000	−4	120,000	−4	115,000
Stelazine	125,000	−4	120,000	−8	110,000	+9	120,000
Total	1,090,000	−4	1,045,000	7	1,120,000	−1	1,110,000

Source: Adapted from Moskowitz (1960).

108

degree of skepticism). What is Librium? When should it be used? What are its limitations? How does it fit into my practice? Please read on . . .

John Kallir, later to become head of his own ad agency, wrote this copy and others that used as a theme a statement from one of the papers published on the drug: "Librium is as different from the tranquilizers as they were from the barbiturates." Another frequently used phrase identified Librium as "the successor to the tranquilizers" (Figure 6.6).

Moskowitz noted that the effect of the new drug was greatest on some of the lesser competition—Atarax and the newly introduced meprobamate analog Striatran. The latter drug, then touted as having significant benefits over its parent compound, might have expected a good future. Librium, however, stole the thunder and Striatran enjoyed one good year in 1961 followed by a terminal decline in use.

The success of Librium did not mean the end of other minor tranquilizers or their advertising. The early 1960s found many products hitting hard at the theme of normalizing living. Miltown (in its long-acting form Meprospan) was supported by a series of case histories. Vistaril added preoperative fear to its list of indications, and Trepidone, too, provided small "slices of life" (Figure 6.7). Nor did Librium fail to promote its use for a better family life.

Advertising Criticism

Almost from the outset, the advertising of the minor tranquilizers (and of prescription drugs in general) was the target of criticism. Some of this criticism has been reported earlier and more will be included in Chapter 9, but additional discussion is appropriate here.

Dowling (1963), in a frequently quoted article in the *Journal of the American Medical Association*, set the stage for a discussion of the use of new drugs by physicians this way:

> The fruits of the labor of thousands of scientists in laboratories, the mountains of data amassed by these and other investigators, the millions of words spawned by the advertising copywriters, all must be beamed to a single spot—to the brain of the individual physician, who must decide whether or not to give a particular drug to a particular patient. Experts may advise, salesmen may cajole, and patients may plead. But the physician must decide.

Although talking of drugs in general, Dowling might well have been referring to the minor tranquilizers when he described the "reprehensible" practice of using a drug in place of a diagnosis. He quoted Matthew Arnold's poem, "The Wish," which describes the physician who gives "the

Librium and the 66 tranquilizers

The era of tranquilizers that preceded Librium therapy saw a long succession of drugs — sixty-six by the latest count. And yet, today Librium is considered by many clinicians as the successor to this entire group. The reasons? The physician can manage *more patients* and control a *wider area* of anxiety-linked symptoms with Librium than with any tranquilizer or group of tranquilizers. Librium is the biggest step yet toward *"pure" anxiety relief* as distinct from central sedative or hypnotic action.

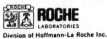
FIGURE 6.6

110

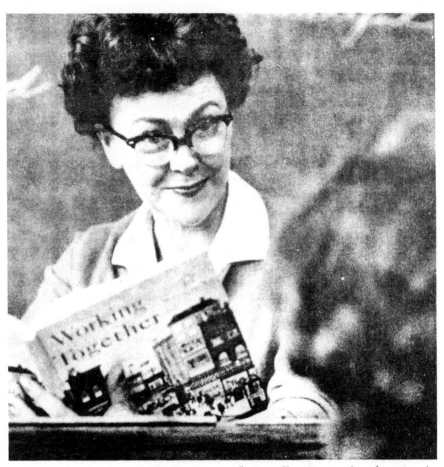

"Notice any change, Mrs. T.?" *Well, Doctor... When I realized that I looked forward to teaching... really enjoyed being with the children again I knew things were better...* "Ever feel light-headed?" *No... not at all. I feel perfectly normal now.*

this could be your "anxiety patient" on

TREPIDONE

MEPHENOXALONE LEDERLE

In the treatment of mild to moderate tension and anxiety, the normalizing effect of TREPIDONE leaves the patient emotionally stable, mentally alert. Adult dose: One 400 mg. tablet, four times daily. Supplied: Half-scored tablets, 400 mg., bottle of 50. Request complete information on indications, dosage, precautions and contraindications from your Lederle representative, or write to Medical Advisory Department.

LEDERLE LABORATORIES, A Division of AMERICAN CYANAMID COMPANY, Pearl River, N. Y.

FIGURE 6.7

ill he cannot cure a name." In a phrase not only well turned but backed by some substantial data, Dowling decried the physicians who "give the ill they cannot name a drug."

How does the physician decide? Katz (1972) followed an imaginary patient through the advertising of various drugs in medical journals in a clever and telling description of the doctor's dilemma.

> Drug A is said to enable the child to surmount the everyday "anxieties of childhood which get out of hand." These may include "school, dental visits and the dark." Drug B will remove the teen-ager's anxieties concerned with going to college. These may include "exposure to new friends, new influences and a newly developed apprehension about unstable national and world conditions." If the problems associated with going off to college prove too much (possibly because drug B wasn't taken) and the adolescent runs away from home, the parents who "failed to communicate" with their offspring can take drug C. If college is survived and the patient is male, drug D will allow him an "emotional breather easing anxiety in the face of continual unavoidable stress of the generation gap, thinning hair, automation, and social pressure which assault the man in the prime of life." If the patient is female drug E is prescribed for the "woman of 35 who has collected a college degree she has never used, children underfoot most of the day" (perhaps because they are not on drug A), "a husband whose career takes him away most of the time" (perhaps he should be on drug D) and "a folder of unpaid bills and various physical symptoms—real or imaginary." Husband or wife might also do well to have a his-and-hers supply of drug F to prevent "excessive anxiety which adversely affects attention and concentration." Assuming that drugs D and F or E and F are not incompatible and the patient survives to the age of 65, drug G may be needed because he or she has an "ailing spouse, a decreased income, grown children seldom seen." Other possibilities include drug H, which may be necessary for the patient to "adjust to old age and make later years productive years," or drug I because she is "widowed and alone (with irritable colon syndrome)." If the patient was so unfortunate as to become ill during his lifetime, he may need drug J "to help clarify the origin of somatic symptoms by relieving the accompanying psychoneurotic anxiety and depression," drug K "to prevent the psychic stress accompanying hospitalization for an illness or operation" or drug L to relieve "the emotional stress that may be detrimental to cardiac function in the cardiac patient who has to be calm."

Hill (1977) was one of many to criticize the use of drugs for the "human problems of living." He cited as an example a Librium ad in a 1969 issue of the *Journal of American College Health Association*. The ad, which showed a worried young college woman, suggested that Librium could "help her get back on her feet" from a situation that might "force her to reevaluate herself and her goals" and become "more sensitive to and apprehensive about material and world conditions."

Stimson (1975b), in his review of psychotropic drug advertisements in England, expressed a variety of concerns, one of which was the tendency, in advertising, to offer a solution to the world's problems. He quoted this passage from a Librium ad as an example:

> The sixties.
> It is ten years since Librium became available. Ten anxious years of aggravation and demonstration, Cuba and Vietnam, assassination and a devaluation, Biafra and Czechoslovakia. Ten turbulent years in which the world-wide climate of anxiety and aggression has given Librium—with its specific calming action and its remarkable safety margin—a unique and still growing role in helping mankind to meet the challenge of a changing world.

Lennard et al. (1970) described the marketing communications of the drug industry as "mystification," i.e., the substitution of false issues for actual issues, in this case, "relabeling an increasing number of human and personal problems as medical problems." They presented evidence of their premise from drug advertisements, which purportedly offered oversimplified answers to complex problems. Indeed, although the drug advertisements were provided as evident and perhaps the cause of the oversimplification, the issue raised by Lennard et al. (1970) is more social than individual, i.e.,

> through the creation of chemical barriers, and through diminishing gross social deviance, drugs may actually serve to perpetuate malignant patterns and social arrangements. Were drugs not so readily available, pressure for other solutions and the pursuit of alternative options might be encouraged.

At a 1971 conference, Robert Dean, a vice president for Smith Kline and French Laboratories, provided a remarkable view of the preparation of drug advertising, especially for psychotropic drugs. Dean reviewed medical dicta from the 1950s concerning the emotionally disturbed patient. He found the emphasis to be on "recognition" of the disturbance, rather than, necessarily, on drug use. Dean said the advertisers read the same material the physician did:

> Meanwhile, back at the advertising departments of the pharmaceutical companies with tranquilizers, copywriters were reading the same articles, seeing the same data. They knew they had drug products that—for some people, for the first time—represented a way to obtain relief from

uncomfortable, even overwhelming symptoms. So copywriters, too, wrote about recognition and then about their product, all the while believing they were doing a good thing.

The ads being made fun of weren't from *my* company, so I can afford a small laugh or two, and I can beg off trying to defend this or that one. Yet they aren't all that different from some of ours. They have this in common: they call attention to emotional problems and anxieties all of us have; they state that most people can live with these by adjusting, adapting, coping; but then, some patients sometimes cannot. They respond with excessive anxiety, and this anxiety may be amenable to treatment with such-and-such a drug.

How do such ads come about? I am not a copywriter, but I may be able to illuminate the "etiology" of an ad for anxiety. First, we should remember that the ads appear in medical journals; they are addressed to physicians only; they are describing *patients*. The people who successfully adjust, adapt, cope aren't coming to the physician, aren't reading the medical journals or magazines (disparaging these magazines by calling them "throw-aways" doesn't change the fact that they are sent only to physicians). One can assume that the anxious or depressed *patient* has come to a physician's office and has thereby selected himself from the rest of us anxious and depressed people, who are presumably coping. The ads deal with—or should be dealing with (I can't vouch for everybody's ads) the anxiety of *disease*, not everyday anxiety. (Dean 1971)

It is unfortunate that the literature on the minor tranquilizers contains little or no additional insight of the type provided by Dean. The workaday activities in advertising and the motives and attitudes of those individuals engaged in them are never revealed. One is left, instead, with the often sinister view provided by the critics of amoral (even immoral?) people seeking chinks in the physician's armor of skepticism through which to thrust a convincing blade of propaganda. The counter view is, one supposes by necessity, couched in carefully weighed legal terms that leave one with the alternative impression that the ads are produced entirely by a computer that checks each word and syllable against an FDA-written guidebook.

Trends in Tranquilizer Advertising

Hundreds of advertisements appeared in support of the various minor tranquilizers. A complete review would be impractical if not impossible. As an alternative systematic approach to surveying such ads, we decided to focus on two journals, *Medical Economics* and the *Journal of the American Medical Association*. Somewhat different approaches were used in each case.

Medical Economics Review

Medical Economics was chosen for inspection because it is a controlled circulation magazine (i.e., sent to physicians without charge), is well known, and contains significant amounts of advertising. The approach used in the *Medical Economics* survey was to review ads for minor tranquilizers appearing in the first issue of each year beginning with the introduction of Valium in 1964. Each ad was read and categorized by the general appeal used. An overview is presented in Table 6.2, with more detail in the narrative that follows. This approach allows, at least, an appreciation for the appeals received by a hypothetical physician who received (and read) these issues.

TABLE 6.2. Minor Tranquilizer Advertising in *Medical Economics*, 1964–81

Year	Total Number of Ads	Product	General Appeals
1964	6	Valium	Introductory ad; strong animal and clinical studies
		Butisol	Reducing the nervous tension of the "nervous personality" (a businessman)
		Atarax	Treatment of more than one member of the family for "communicable anxiety"
		Deprol	Anxiety associated with depression
		Miltown	Versatility across all patients
		Meprospan	Somatic complaints, long acting
1965	7	Valium	The "Somatic Mask"—use in chest pain
		Meprospan	Same as 1964
		Deprol	Same as 1964
		Miltown	Cardiovascular disease
		Equanil	Anxiety, alone or with somatic condition
		Atarax	Preoperative tension
		Vistaril	Calm the "animal brain"

TABLE 6.2 *(continued)*

Year	Total Number of Ads	Product	General Appeals
1966	4	Valium	"Somatic Mask"—use in epigastric pain
		Miltown	Years of experience; a standard therapy
		Vistaril	Alcoholism
		Atarax	Geriatric syndrome
1967	5	Valium	Heartburn/epigastric distress
		Miltown	Broad usefulness
		Meprobamate (generic)	Lower price
		Vistaril	Alcoholism
		Atarax	Same as 1966
1968	5	Valium	Somatic conditions
		Librium	Tablet dosage form
		Miltown (1)	Computer Age Compulsion
		Miltown (2)	Battered Parent Syndrome
		Vistaril	Alcoholism
1969	6	Valium	Muscle spasm
		Librium	Anxiety
		Deprol	Chronic illness
		Vistaril	Geriatric anxiety
		Butisol	Daytime sedation
		Serax	Anxiety associated with somatic illness (?)
1970	4	Valium	Gastrointestinal symptoms
		Librium	General anxiety
1971	5	Valium	Spastic gut
		Librium	Postmyocardial infarction
		Serax	Work-related tension
		Deprol	Geriatric anxiety-depression
		Meprospan	Same as 1970
1972	2	Valium	Postcoronary tension
		Miltown	Reminder
1973	4	Valium	Gastrointestinal disease
		Librium	Postcoronary tension
		Miltown	Experience, predictability
		Atarax	Cardiac patients
1974	4	Valium	Muscle relaxant
		Librium	Cardiac problems
		Vistaril	Cardiac problems

TABLE 6.2 *(continued)*

Year	Total Number of Ads	Product	General Appeals
		Atarax	Allergic dermatitis
1975	2	Valium	Psychic tension
		Librium	Cardiac problems
1976	2	Valium	Muscle relaxant
		Librium	Concomitant use with other drugs
1977	3	Valium	Multiple uses
		Librium	Predictable response
		Atarax	Allergic dermatosis with anxiety
1978	5	Valium	Psychic tension in hypertension
		Vistaril	Cardiac patients
		Verstran	Versatile dosage
		Ativan	Pharmacokinetic profile
		Azene	Option to other benzodiazepines
1979	3	Valium	Psychotherapeutic/muscle relaxant
		Ativan	Simple metabolism
		Tranxene	Lack of sedation
1980	6	Valium	Multiple uses
		Librium	General anxiety/ dependability
		Tranxene	Lack of sedation
		Ativan (1)	Importance of pharmacokinetic profile
		Ativan (2)	Lack of long-acting metabolites
		Ativan (3)	Gastrointestinal problems
1981	5	Valium	Institutional
		Librium	General performance
		Ativan	Same as (1) in 1980
		Tranxene	Lack of withdrawal effects
		Centrax	Few side effects

The year 1964 saw the introduction of Valium to the medical profession—and the world. Valium was to be used for "situational, stress-induced nervous tension, the psychic tension of the common psycho-neuroses," and tension that was intensified by somatic components.

Eight pages of advertising was devoted to the new product. Comparisons were made of its effects in "vicious rats" and "vicious monkeys" with meprobamate and with chlorpromazine. Clinical studies, according to the ad, had already involved more than 25,000 patients. Among those who benefited were business executives, those suffering from tension "due to stressful interfamily relationships," fearful and pessimistic elderly, premenstrual tension sufferers, and victims of dermatologic disorders.

The advertisement was free of dramatic illustration—rather it resembled, and indeed was, a clinical report complete with ten references, all of them published. No mention was made of Librium, although Valium was described as the "latest in the series of Roche-discovered benzodiazepine compounds."

Physicians reading the rest of that issue of Medical Economics would find five additional ads for products to treat anxiety. Butisol, though not strictly a tranquilizer, was often used for anxiety and was promoted for the "nervous personality." Atarax was part of an ad in which it was suggested by copy and illustration that an elderly person living with a family might communicate her anxiety such that she ("the intruder") and other members of the "resentful family" might all need Atarax. Wallace Laboratories offered three advertisements. Deprol was supported by the female patient complaining, "I can't cope any more. . . . The kids drive me crazy. I worry about everything . . . feel exhausted all the time." Elsewhere, Wallace told the physician that "Miltown is helpful in almost every aspect of daily practice. Virtually any of your patients can be given the drug either as a primary treatment or as an adjunct to other therapy." (Indeed, meprobamate had been combined with a number of other drugs, including dextroamphetamine, conjugated estrogens, analgesics, and, in Deprol, benactyzine.) Thirteen different kinds of patients were shown in photographs to emphasize the drug's versatility. Finally, Wallace offered Meprospan, its sustained-release Miltown, with twice-a-day dosage.

In 1965, one year after its introduction, Valium was suggested for use when the "classic signs of cardiac disease" were found to be, in fact, a "Somatic Mask." This Mask was defined as a "psychophysiologic equivalent of psychic tension." Six other antianxiety agent advertisements appeared in the same issue. Wallace was back with its Deprol and Meprospan ads. Miltown was suggested (as was Valium) for the "emotional factors in cardiovascular disease." The competing meprobamate, Equanil, was promoted to "help . . . anxious patients through periods of stress." Both Atarax and Vistaril were also advertised. Both are hydroxyzine and both are sold by divisions of Pfizer, but the former drug was suggested for preoperative fear (as well as "every degree of anxiety in patients under 6 to over 60"). Whereas the ad for the latter instructed the physician that the "animal brain" (limbic system) was the seat of human emotions and the site of Vistaril action.

In 1966, the Somatic Mask was one cause of epigastric pain. Valium was the suggested means of intervention in a cycle that including situational conflicts, somatic complaints, and psychic tensions. Miltown was cited for its "eminent role in medical practice" and photographically shown in the company of such standards as pencillin, digitalis, cortisone, aspirin, and vitamins. Pfizer, having completed its education of the physicians about the limbic system, said of Vistaril, "Its site of action is the seat of anxiety." In promoting its use in alcoholism, Pfizer noted that Vistaril had fewer side effects and complications than the diazepines, phenothiazines, or meprobamate. Its sister product, Atarax, was being promoted for the "geriatric syndrome."

In 1967, Valium continued its Somatic Mask theme in heartburn and epigastric pressure, while both Vistaril and Atarax advertising also followed the pattern of the previous year. The makers of Miltown challenged doctors to "name a disorder in which 'Miltown' has *not* been used to ease accompanying anxiety." Wallace pointed to its widespread use for either primary or secondary diagnosis and emphasized its more than a decade of use. Any physician with the temerity to suggest a use not cited in the literature was offered a woodcut print of a famous medical figure.

Looking over the Wallace shoulder in the same issue was McKesson Laboratories. McKesson advertised their generic meprobamate in one of the earliest ads featuring the possibility of savings through generic prescribing.

In 1968, Roche described galvanic skin resistance to explain the relationship between stress and somatic responses and to promote Valium. Valium's older-sister product, Librium, was now announced to be available in tablets as "Libritabs." Miltown introduced two new "syndromes of the 1960s," the Computer Age Compulsion and the Battered Parent Syndrome. "Whenever human emotions become folded, spindled and multilated—Miltown can frequently be of help." Vistaril, meanwhile, was demonstrating, by graph, its superiority to Librium in alcoholism treatment.

The 1969 Valium ad introduced a new indication for use, muscle spasm. This allowed Roche the opportunity to reemphasize the antianxiety properties of Librium. Wallace suggested that Deprol might be useful in helping chronically ill patients cope with their disease and treatment, and Butisol was offered for the housewife who was shown, bound in ropes, by her child. The wording foreshadowed criticism and, ultimately, FDA action: "The 'daytime sedative' for everyday situational stress. When stress is situational-environmental pressure, worry over illness—the treatment often calls for an anxiety-allaying agent." Vistaril was now being promoted for geriatric anxiety, and Pfizer was pointing out that "this product is not subject to the Drug Abuse Control Amendments." A new benzodiazepine, Serax, by Wyeth, also appeared. The advertisement was so low key as to sound quite unlike a promotional effort: "Anxiety and tension stemming from organic illness may undermine your patient's cooperation and possibly retard success of primary therapy. If his emotional symptoms persist in the face of your counsel and reassurance, you may want to consider adjunctive use of Serax."

The 1970 Valium ad, one of a series, portrayed the doctoral candidate with a thesis to finish, persistent indigestion, and a normal gastrointestinal series and physical examination. Although definitely taken out of context, one sentence is intriguing. "For this kind of patient—with no demonstrable pathology—consider the usefulness of Valium." In the same issue, Roche was giving physicians (or Pfizer) a real lesson on the limbic system. Mostly about cats, this ad for Librium nevertheless left the strong impression that Librium and limbic were somehow associated for the good of the patient. Meanwhile, McNeil was announcing an "old drug"—Butisol. "If just discovered," the ad read, "Butisol Sodium might well be the exciting new 'tranquilizer' of 1970." Wallace, on the other hand, used the King of Hearts to emphasize that Miltown, too (as Meprospan), could help the heart patient.

"When psychic tension aggravates G.I. disorders," Valium could help, according to the 1971 ad. Librium, on the other hand, was indicated for the post-heart attack patient whose family has convinced him he may never work again. That was not the problem of the prospective Serax patient, who had too much work to do. If Serax could help him stop worrying about the work, maybe he would be able to do some of it. Vistaril, in 1971, was indicated for the anxious insomniac, Deprol for the geriatric patient, and the King of Hearts was back to speak for Meprospan.

In 1972, Valium was the Roche choice for the postcoronary patient, a position occupied by Librium the year before. Miltown was a reminder only. The next year, it was back to Librium for the postcoronary patient, while Valium was promoted for gastrointestinal disease. The "enduring value of Miltown" in 1973 was pictorially associated with Stonehenge ("Alone, monolithic purpose confirmed"), as Wallace suggested that with "proper patient selection" (not defined or described), patient response was predictable. Atarax was back with the cardiac patient as its target.

In 1974, Roche, using a technique that was to occur frequently in its promotion, employed an animal model (cat) to describe a "possible mode and site of action" of Valium as a muscle relaxant. Librium was promoted to allay the anxiety of the cardiac patient who had no organic problem. Vistaril was advertised for virtually the same patients as Librium, but

Atarax used a dramatic illustration to suggest the existence of a cycle of anxiety and allergic/dermatologic disorder that could affect an entire family. An eye-catching photograph of a mother and her two children (apparently) naked served to attract the reader's attention.

Only Valium and Librium were advertised in the 1975 issue. In the Valium advertisement, Roche identified three types of individuals who suffered from psychic tension: those who could handle it without medical help; those who needed the physician's reassurance and support; and those who needed reassurance, counseling, and Valium.

The Valium ad is notable for the way in which it explained the role of the minor tranquilizer: "While Valium (diazepam) will relieve most kinds of psychic tension it *isn't* for common tensions of everyday life—tight schedules, traffic jams, final exams. Although these tensions may bother people, most cope with them very well." The ad went even further. "It *isn't* even for many of the tensions and anxieties people complain about. For example, those due to the normal fear and apprehensions about an illness o diagnostic procedure or surgery."

The fact that the theme of this advertisement was almost certainly a response to FDA pressure (see Chapter 9) does not minimize its remarkable character. Precautions had long been included in the "small-print" prescribing information of minor tranquilizer ads, but here was the leader saying openly that Valium was not for everything.

Librium, in the same issue, was suggested as an adjunct to counseling and reassurance for the cardiovascular patient. Its relative safety for use concomitantly with other drugs (with the possible exception of anticoagulants) was also emphasized. The use of Librium with a range of other drugs was the major theme of the 1976 ad, while Valium was promoted for muscle spasms.

In 1977, the broad range of indications of Valium was highlighted, while Librium was called "anxiety specific" and attention directed to its predictability based on years of use. Atarax was back with the added claim of antihistaminic activity for use in allergic dermatoses.

The old Somatic Mask of Valium advertisements was subtly reintroduced in the 1978 ad, which suggested its use in the distressed hypertensive patient. The ad was notable for its use of a black model—a relative rarity in drug advertising. Vistaril was promoted for the "clinical" and "excessive" anxiety of the cardiac patient.

Three new drugs were also advertised in the 1978 issue of *Medical Economics*. New Verstran provided both the effectiveness of benzodiazepines and dosage versatility (the "versatile tranquilizer"). The "versatility" was provided via a 10-milligram tablet that could be broken in half. The "Ativan Experience" was never defined, but the drug was described as "strikingly effective in the symptomatic relief of anxiety neuroses and transient situational disturbances." Efforts to set Ativan apart from other benzodiazepines involved in introduction of pharmacokinetic concepts. Endo, apparently lacking anything remarkable to say about its new Azene, described it as the "option" benzodiazepine and illustrated the ad with pick-up sticks.

In 1979, Valium was described as the only drug with the two distinct effects of psychotherapeutic and skeletal muscle relaxant. This was perhaps a reminder to the reader that all benzodiazepines were not alike, at least in terms of FDA-approved indications. Ativan advertising took a somewhat different approach, showing that Tranxene, Verstran, Valium, and Librium were all ultimately metabolized to desmethyl-diazepam and oxazepam, whereas Ativan was not. The ad also footnoted that these products, excluding Ativan, were Category IV Drug Enforcement Agency (DEA) agents. Tranxene was offered as a tranquilizer without excessive sedating properties.

Roche returned, in 1980, to its promotion of Valium as unique in its range of clinical indications and dosage forms. The Librium themes were familiar as well—predictability, long experience, safe concomitant use— and Tranxene continued to emphasize a lack of sedation. Ativan was supported in the 1980 issue by three different ads. In the largest, the pharmacokinetic profile was again highlighted as a reason for choosing Ativan over the other six benzodiazepines available. A second ad elaborated on this theme, referring to an article in the *New England Journal of Medicine* that expressed concern about long-acting metabolites of benzodiazepines. The third ad simply suggested use of Ativan for anxiety in patients with gastrointestinal complaints.

1981 saw Roche offering a monograph on the benzodiazepines by John Marks and an institutional ad for Librium. In the latter case, the "greatness" of Librium was compared with the fate of the Edsel (shown in the pictures), which was introduced at about the same time. The pharmacokinetic Ativan ad was repeated, while Tranxene was said to "taper gently" when treatment concluded. The primary "pitch" for the latest benzodiazepine, Centrax, was a low order of side effects.

Journal of the American Medical Association Review

The *Journal of the American Medical Association* study was an attempt to determine if drug advertising had promoted the use of minor tranquilizers for "problems of living" and whether such promotion continues at present.*

---

*Some of the materials in this section were previously published as Gray and Smith (1984).

The objectives of this study were the following:

1. To determine if appeals found in ads for minor tranquilizers in a sample of medical journal advertisements have changed through the years, and the direction of such change.
2. To determine and compare the frequency of utilization of appeals by both headline/illustration and text.
3. To determine and compare chronologically, through the years 1968–81, the frequency of appeals by both headline/illustration and text.
4. To determine and compare the number and frequency of the appearance of appeals promoting minor tranquilizers as cures for "problems of living."

Data were collected from the *Journal of the American Medical Association*. This journal was selected because it is the official publication of the AMA, is one of relatively few paid subscription medical journals, was convenient for research, and reaches all medical specialties. It is recognized that different advertising strategies may be employed in different media, especially those directed to psychiatrists.

Initially, the study was to span a 25-year period from 1955 to 1980. However, prior to 1968, advertisements were not bound along with the body of the journals at the University of Mississippi library. (Several other libraries were contacted regarding the ads to no avail.) Issues of the journal for analysis were chosen at random. A 25 percent sample was obtained, randomly selecting an issue from among the first four issues of each year under study and then selecting each fourth issue. A total of 257 ads, unique ads, repeats, and percentages, for minor tranquilizers were identified during the 14-year period January 1968 through December 1981. The identification of minor tranquilizers for study was taken from the American Medical Association Drug Evaluations, Category 6.28, "minor tranquilizers." A list of all drugs identified within the sample and the approximate year of introduction to the market can be found in Table 6.3.

Content analysis was utilized to identify and categorize all the appeals of the ads under study. Headline/illustration and text were categorized separately. Single ads could have multiple appeals. A total of 14 specific categories was developed. These categories were further collected into five broad groups: Generalized Anxiety, Anxiety Associated with Disease, Treatment of a Condition, Problems of Living, and Other Appeals.

The headline/illustration was considered as one item for purposes of analysis. The appeal or appeals of each headline/illustration were recorded in the approriate category. For example, if the headline/illustration referred to anxiety related to cardiovascular disease, it was recorded as "Cardiovascular" appeal. The content of the text was recorded in the same manner. All distinct appeals were recorded.

The content analysis was conducted to determine the degree to which the appeal of Problems of Living, among others, has been used in advertising the minor tranquilizers. We were also interested in examining changes in the proportionate uses of the respective appeals over time.

The numbers of ads—original ads, repeat ads, total ads, and percentages—by drug are exhibited in Table 6.3. Ads for 14 different drugs were identified as part of our sample. The drugs are ranked in decreasing order of frequency of appearance of the original, unique ads. Librium and Valium were the most frequently advertised drugs within our sample. These two drugs represent 61.9 percent of all advertisements studied.

The total number and percentage of appeals by scientific category and general category are shown in Table 6.4. This table represents only original ads, excluding repeats.

The largest specific appeal category was category A (Generalized Anxiety), followed by category B (Cardiovascular Disease). Category I (Problems of Living) had a total of 13 appeals, or 3.8 percent, and was the seventh largest category (tied with J—Animal Studies). Thus, Problems of Living appear to represent a very small number of appeals found in ads for minor tranquilizers.

The five general categories represented by Table 6.4 rank as follows: Anxiety Associated with Disease, Generalized Anxiety, Treatment of a Condition, Other Appeals, and Problems of Living. Thus, this information indicates that advertising appeals directed toward problems of living were represented in a very small number of ads. Approximately, one-third of all studied appeals were directed toward Anxiety Associated with Disease, either anxiety resulting from disease or clinical condition or anxiety as a factor in somatic disease. Sixty-two percent of all appeals were directed toward either Anxiety Associated with Disease or Generalized Anxiety.

The Generalized Anxiety appeal has remained fairly consistent through the years. Of the Anxiety Associated with Disease appeals, most occurred in 1969 and none in 1975 and 1981. This appeal was prevalent in the years 1969–74.

Of the appeals associated with Treatment of a Condition, most occurred in the year 1970, and none appeared in the years 1973, 1976, and 1978. (Overall, this appeal seems to have been fairly consistent, discounting the high-appearance year and the three low-appearance years.) All of the Problems of Living appeals occurred in the years 1969–72 in headline/illustration. Two appeals were noted in both 1969 and 1970 and one appeal each in 1971 and 1972. During the years surveyed, the Problems of Living appeals were not widely used in headline/illustration, and such appeals have not appeared at all since 1972. Of the Other Appeals category, one-

TABLE 6.3. Total Number of Ads—Original and Repeats by Drug

	Year Introduced to Market	Number of Original Ads	Percentage	Number of Repeat Ads	Percentage	Number of Total Ads	Percentage of Total Ads
Librium	1960	46	35.7	42	32.8	88	34.2
Valium	1962	44	34.1	27	21.1	71	27.7
Tranxene	1972	7	5.4	15	11.7	22	8.5
Serax	1965	4	3.1	16	12.5	20	7.8
Atarax	1956	5	3.9	5	3.9	10	3.9
Vistaril	1958	4	3.1	6	4.7	10	3.9
Miltown	1955	4	3.1	6	4.7	10	3.9
Ativan	1977	4	3.1	3	2.3	7	2.7
Meprospan	1958	2	1.6	4	3.1	6	2.3
Azene	1977	2	1.6	3	2.3	5	1.9
Equanil	1955	3	2.3	0	0.0	3	1.2
Verstran	1977	2	1.6	1	0.8	3	1.2
Sk-Bamate	1971	1	0.8	0	0.0	1	0.4
Xanax	1981	1	0.8	0	0.0	1	0.4
Total		129	100.0	128	100.0	257	100.0

TABLE 6.4. Total Number of Appeals by Type

Appeal Category	Definition	Headline/Illustration		Text		Total	
		Number	Percentage	Number	Percentage	Number	Percentage
A	Generalized Anxiety	39	27.1	56	29.0	95	28.2
	Subtotal	39	27.1	56	29.0	95	28.2
Anxiety Associated with							
B	Cardiovascular Disease	28	19.4	35	18.1	63	18.7
C	Gastrointestinal Disease Unspecified	15	10.4	22	11.4	37	10.9
E	Psychosomatic Diseae	1	0.7	9	4.7	10	2.9
K	Arthritis Unspecified Organic	1	0.7	1	0.5	2	0.6
M	Disease	1	0.7	1	0.5	2	0.6
	Subtotal	46	31.1	68	35.2	114	33.8
Treatment of							
D	Allergies/Dermatological Problems	5	3.5	5	2.6	10	2.9
F	Alcoholism	2	1.4	3	1.6	5	1.5
G	Insomnia	4	2.8	10	5.2	14	4.1
H	Muscle Spasms	17	11.8	18	9.3	35	10.3
	Subtotal	28	19.4	36	18.7	64	19.1
I	Problems of Living	6	4.2	7	3.6	13	3.8
	Subtotal	6	4.2	7	3.6	13	3.8
Other Appeals							
J	Animal Studies	5	3.5	8	4.1	13	3.8
L	Clinical/Research	17	11.8	16	8.3	33	9.8
N	Miscellaneous	3	2.1	2	1.0	5	1.5
	Subtotal	25	17.4	26	13.5	51	15.1
Total		144	100.0	193	100.0	337	100.0

sixth occurred in 1981 and none in 1968 and 1979. This appeal category, which includes safety, efficiency, and clinical resarch, seems to be consistent during the time under study, at least in headline/illustration.

Appeals found in the text of advertisements rank as follows: Anxiety Associated with Disease, Generalized Anxiety, Treatment of a Condition, Other Appeals, and Problems of Living. Appeals identified in the text rank by frequency in the same order as those identified in headline/illustration: The number of appeals found in the text is generally greater than those found in headline/illustration owing to more multiple appeals in individual ads.

The Generalized Anxiety appeals occurred frequently in the years 1969, 1972, 1970, 1974, and 1981. This appeal seemed to be identified consistently through the years.

Of the Anxiety Associated with a Disease appeals, most occurred in the years 1969–72 and 1974. (This appeal has decreased since the early 1970s.) The Treatment of a Condition appeal occurred most frequently in 1970 and was not used in 1973 or 1976. As indicated in Table 6.4, the Problems of Living appeal again occurred in the years 1969 through 1972 with one exception: One such appeal was identified in the text of an ad in 1980. The Other Appeal category occurred more frequently in 1973–75 and 1981.

Based on the results reported here, it would appear that the use of minor tranquilizers for problems of living is no longer utilized in any significant way as a promotional theme. It is notable that this appeal essentially disappeared from the *Journal of the American Medical Association* after 1973. It seems likely that this was a direct result of intervention by the FDA.

The FDA finds itself in a difficult regulatory position when drugs are prescribed for social problems. In 1971, the administration sent a letter to advertisers of psychotropic drugs asking them to cancel promotions that suggested the use of the drugs for everyday or minor life stresses. FDA officials reported that the response was positive (Simmons 1974). Dr. Henry Simmons, former director of the FDA Bureau of Drugs, noted that safety and efficacy considerations do not support the use of psychoactive drugs for coping with nonpathological personal and interpersonal problems. He also pointed out that drug advertising problems are manifestations of the existence of an attitude that such use is appropriate.

Although a cause-and-effect relationship can not be supported, one coincidence is striking. The year 1973, after which use of the Problems of Living appeal disappeared from our sample, was followed in two years by the first overall sales decline in minor tranquilizers, a decline that has continued (Chapter 4).

Interestingly, the appeal category that appeared most frequently was use of these drugs for Anxiety Associated with Organic Illness. This appeal, too, has been criticized.

Hemminki (1974a) reported that the prominent use of psychotropic drugs in somatic diseases may be a factor in increased psychotropic drug use. Her comments on possible reasons for such use are thought-provoking:

> The psychosomatic concept, that much in somatic diseases is a reflection of psychic disturbances, may offer an explanation for the abundant use of psychotropic drugs; the therapy has been no more than of derisory nature. It might be responsible as an expression of incompetence: the doctor, incapable of applying other therapeutical means, prescribes a drug, on this occasion a psychotropic one.

We believe that the "derisory" charge may be overdrawn, although perhaps not totally unjustified. There is adequate specific therapy for most of the organic (somatic) conditions for which minor tranquilizers ads suggest treatment. In fact, use of these drugs is usually concomitant with other therapy in such cases. The legitimacy of relieving anxiety while a physiologic condition is treated is an issue that cannot be resolved here, although there is considerable literature to support the practice. Finally, it could be argued that the General Anxiety appeal is similar to the Problems of Living appeal. Nevertheless, the latter is specific in nature, is the most frequent target of criticism, and clearly represents areas of human conflict that cannot be resolved through drug use. General anxiety is admittedly amorphous but does, at least, admit to physician judgment in selecting drug therapy. Appeals in the Problems of Living category imply that scientific difficulties in the home or in the workplace are amenable to drug therapy.

SUMMARY

The information that physicians received about the minor tranquilizers, through their medical journals especially, has varied considerably over the years. This is true whether the source was their colleagues or drug company promotion. Both were characterized by early, perhaps unwarranted enthusiasm. As the drug class matured, the professional literature became more critical. Indeed, a rather general view of articles by physicians follows the curve shown in Chapter 1 of early enthusiasm; harsh, sometimes strident criticism; followed by a balanced view of the benefits and hazards of the use of these drugs.

The promotional literature, too, has achieved greater balance, although that balance seems to have been reached at least in part through the encouragement of more stringent FDA advertising regulations. More background on these developments is provided in Chapter 9.

7

SOCIAL ISSUES

> "The solicitor pays for his groceries by
> giving legal advice to the grocer, the
> grocer pays for his medicines by supply-
> ing sugar to the chemist—and so on."
> Edmund Crispin
> *Beware of Trains*

THE ROLE OF SOCIAL SCIENTISTS

It seems unlikely that any single class of drugs in the medical care system has been laden with the social baggage that accompanies the minor tranquilizers. Individual drugs (dimethysulfoxide, thalidomide, Laetrile) have captured the public fancy or aroused the public ire, but the minor tranquilizers, from their very beginnings, brought social issues that have yet to be resolved. Unfortunately, as we shall see, the medical professionals charged with the administration of the drugs have received surprisingly little assistance from the social scientists who might have offered it.

The minor tranquilizers were a part of that special kind of phenomenon that Stolley (1971) and others have referred to as "cultural lag." The drugs arrived long before the social scientists were apparently able to deal with them. This is unfortunate, since physicians, especially the general practitioners, might have benefited from the results of sound research on what society expected of these new drugs and the physicians who prescribed them.

With the exception of study in the context of frank drug abuse, which occupied social scientists through the 1960s and into the 1970s, the minor tranquilizers were (and indeed continue to be) largely ignored by sociologists. This can be viewed only as a phenomenal oversight, given their widespread use and social importance.

The minor tranquilizers have not been totally overlooked by the social scientists, however. Among the social themes developed during their first 25 years have been

- The medicalization of social problems
- Pharmacological Calvinism
- The imbalance of use by women over men
- Drug abuse/addiction

The final item in this list is also a medical problem and is so considered in this book.

Sociologists have engaged themselves somewhat in the study of other issues relating to the minor tranquilizers, and these are dealt with in various places. In this chapter, we will address some of them briefly and the first three of the above in some detail.

Before doing that, however, it must be recognized that the minor tranquilizers certainly inherited some preexisting concern about the potential of drugs to control minds and societies. A number of authors, notably, Aldous Huxley in *Brave New World*, had fictionally suggested an existence at least partially ordered by drugs.*

One of the most arresting comments about the widespread use of psychoactive drugs come from Hammond and Joyce (1975):

> We . . . need to know how drugs influence the judgment *of* the drugged, *about* the drugged, and arising from *interaction* of the drugged with others. How much of our present legislation and other political activity represents interaction modified by such means? Is it better or worse for having been initiated in smoke-filled rooms and wine-filled brains? How many of our future, perhaps present, legislators are experienced users of social drugs other than alcohol and tobacco, and how much difference does this make to their decisions on matters other than drugs?

Lennard et al. (1967) in the mid-1960s raised important issues about the effect of tranquilizer use, not only on the drug taker but also on those with whom he or she normally interacts. They noted five aspects to the subject:

---

*Incredibly, Wallace Laboratories, the producer of Miltown, marketed in the 1950s a muscle relaxant under the brand name Soma, the name of the drug so chillingly involved in Huxley's novel.

1. What is the effect of the drug on the individual?
2. How do other persons change their behavior toward the drug taker?
3. If one member of a group takes a psychoactive drug, does this change the structure and process of the group?
4. How do the characteristics of the group interact with the drug taking?
5. Do group members perceive changes in behavior of a "drugged" individual?

In their experimental study, using a major tranquilizer, some effects on group interaction were noted and the researchers "advance[d] the suggestion that minor interactional deficits and behavior redistribution may exert a major impact on the functioning of social groups." Without criticizing the study, it should be noted that "normal" people received major tranquilizers. In "real life," that would not be likely to happen. That observation notwithstanding, the implication that behavioral change in an individual may have a "ripple effect" in various social groups is extremely important.

In 1971, at one of scores of similar conferences organized during that time to discuss the social implications of drug use, Jacobs voiced the concern that had been voiced many times before and since by others in various ways:

One must consider the broader implications of a culture in which tens of millions of adult citizens have come to use psychoactive drugs to alter virtually every facet of their waking (and sleeping) behavior. What does this say about the impact of modern technology on our style of life? What changes may be evolving in our value system?

Marks (1972) later noted that

there are socially acceptable diseases and socially acceptable drugs with no rational basis for the division, and in our current social pattern the neurosis and psychotropic drugs are still largely socially unacceptable— tolerated as a necessary evil rather than lauded as a great good. Society's approach to neurotic ill health is still broadly "shake yourself out of it."

THE MEDICALIZATION OF HUMAN PROBLEMS

The idea that the minor tranquilizers are used as part of a model that medicalizes problems that are essentially social or human is one that has followed these drugs since their early days on the market. It appears elsewhere in this book, and often.

An example is the work of Koumjian (1981), who suggests that the medicalization of anxiety and tension results from the following attitudes and beliefs supporting the use of Valium: (1) the individualization of anxiety; (2) a reductional view of nonspecific or psychosomatic symptoms; and (3) a belief that Valium has a specific effect in reducing anxiety without inducing any significantly undesirable changes in physiology, social interaction, or subjective experience. Commercial promotion and the characteristics of medical practice are cited by Koumjian as the major reasons for these views.

How did this begin?

Silverman et al. (1981) noted that "psychosocial problems and psychosomatic complaints became legitimized as treatable illnesses simply because there were now new drugs to treat them." They quoted medical sociologist Irving Zola: "By the very acceptance of a specific behavior as an 'illness' and the definition of illness as an undesirable state, the issue becomes not *whether* to deal with a specific problem but *how* and *when*."

Rogers, writing in a 1971 issue of *Psychology Today*, described drug abuse as "Just What the Doctor Ordered." According to him,

> Physicians who overuse psychoactive drugs are wedded to an obsolete medical model of human behavior—the concept that psychological problems have medical causes. This viewpoint widens physicians' jurisdiction by classifying more and more persons as potential medical patients, and it allows an earnest medical healer to respond to all who seek his help.

Who cares about how many psychotropic drugs are used? As Cooperstock (1978b) has observed, there is more than intellectual curiosity involved: "Opposition to reliance on psychotropics for individual solutions to problems of living is a value-laden position." The vigor with which such values are held is shown by her quotation from Lennard and Bernstein (1974):

> There is hardly any doubt that professionals, through their expansion of psychiatric conceptualization to include anxiety, unhappiness, conflict and tension as symptoms of mental disease, have themselves contributed greatly to the very psychic distress they seek to pacify through drugs. Both mental health professionals and the pharmaceutical industry have, by promoting drug taking, promoted a model that has contributed significantly to the medicalization and technocratization of human existence.

The very drugs that appeared (and still appear) to offer physicians promising means of therapy sometimes seemed to divide them. Are psychiatrists physicians (i.e., following a medical model)? Or are they just one of many occupational groups working in the field of mental health?

An especially interesting insight was provided by Dorsey (1975). He cited Gardos's description of the division in psychiatry between those who regard themselves primarily as physicians and those who reject the medical model in favor of alliance with other mental health professionals.

The arrival of the minor tranquilizers and the subsequent successes must be due, at least in part, to the shortage or uneven distribution of psychiatrists, an issue that was explored in an interesting fashion by Koran (1979). Koran compared the psychiatrist distribution with that of lawyers, presented several schemes for improving it, and made the interesting observation that, in 1974, the federal research investment in mental illness was about $40 per person affected, compared with about $200 per person affected in cancer research.

PHARMACOLOGICAL CALVINISM

The concept of pharmacological Calvinism is best understood in the context of the data obtained through the national study of attitudes toward and use of various psychotropic drugs, which has been described in Chapter 4. Without question, the most important and extensive study of the attitudes and beliefs of the public toward tranquilizers and the conditions for which they are used was conducted in collaboration between the Institute for Research in Social Behavior (Berkeley), the Social Research Group of George Washington University, and the Psychopharmacology Research Branch of the NIMH (Manheimer et al. 1973).

Data were collected in late 1970 and early 1971 from a carefully selected sample of 2,552 individuals aged 18–74 years and representing a cross-section of noninstitutionalized American adults. Personal interviews lasting between one and one and one-half hours were used.

The first finding of this survey was that most respondents knew what a tranquilizer was. Only 11 percent said they did not, and almost 70 percent explicitly mentioned the tranquilizer effect. There were differences by type of respondent, however. Nearly one-fourth of those over age 60 did not know what a tranquilizer was; education levels affected this response as well.

Those respondents who knew what a tranquilizer was were asked whether they agreed or disagreed with a range of statements reflecting attitudes and beliefs about tranquilizers. (The number of eligible respondents was now 2,241.) The statements were introduced by the interviewer as follows:

Now, I'm going to give you a list of statements people have made about tranquilizers—that is, pills such as Miltown, Equanil, and Librium that can be used to calm you down or keep you from getting nervous or upset. As you read each statement, please ... tell whether you agree strongly, agree, disagree, or disagree strongly. (Manheimer et al. 1973)

The statements, along with a general measure of responses, are shown in Table 7.1.

The researchers concluded that "it appears that Americans believe tranquilizers are effective but have serious doubts about the morality of using them and about their physical safety." They noted that these views are not unanimous, with the educational level of the respondent being inversely associated with the degree to which respondents associated tranquilizer usage with moral weakness.

Semiprojective techniques were next used to approach respondent attitudes. Respondents were asked to choose an appropriate level of distress for use of either a tranquilizer or an antidepressant. The question was posed as follows:

Let's assume that someone has a supply of pills on hand that a doctor prescribed and said to take as needed. These pills calm you down or make you feel more relaxed (or These pills make you feel more energetic or alert, or lift your spirits). Just suppose that the person is trying to decide whether to take one in each of the following situations. Do you agree or disagree that it's all right to take a pill or medicine like this when someone:

1. is generally doing a good job at work but wants to be relaxed (or to have more energy) in order to be even more efficient and productive?
2. is upset and nervous (or is down in the dumps or has little energy) and not working as he should?
3. is so upset or nervous (or is so depressed or has so little energy) that he is not even able to go to work?
4. wants to relax (or wants more energy) in order to enjoy his family more than usual?
5. is nervous and upset (or is depressed) and can't get along with his family as well as usual?
6. is so upset and nervous (or is so depressed or has so little energy) that he is making life miserable for his family? (Manheimer et al. 1973)

TABLE 7.1. Percentages Agreeing and Disagreeing with Statements Reflecting General Attitudes and Beliefs about Tranquilizers (*n* = 2,241)*

Statement	Agree	Disagree	No Answer/ Don't Know
Efficacy			
Tranquilizers work very well to make a person more calm and relaxed.	74	20	6
Self-awareness and problem solving			
Tranquilizers don't really cure anything; they just cover up the real trouble.	69	25	5
Using tranquilizers just prevents people from working out their problems for themselves.	57	37	6
Self-reliance and strength of character			
It is better to use willpower to solve problems than it is to use tranquilizers.	87	10	3
Taking tranquilizers is a sign of weakness.	40	55	5
Control and responsibility			
Tranquilizers cause people to lose some control over what they do.	61	31	7
Tranquilizers can change your mood so that you just don't care about anything.	66	28	6

Short-term side effects			
One big advantage of tranquilizers is that they *don't* make a person sleepy or groggy.	12	79	9
Tranquilizers often have bad side effects—such as making a person very sleepy or sick to the stomach.	73	18	9
Long-term adverse effects			
Long-term use of tranquilizers may cause real physical harm to your body.	80	14	6
One good thing about tranquilizers is that people do *not* get addicted to them.	18	74	9
Consumer concerns			
Tranquilizers often get on the market before they are thoroughly tested to be sure they are safe.	57	30	12
Tranquilizers are too new for doctors to know what harm they might do to a person.	39	52	9
Many doctors prescribe tranquilizers more than they should.	59	30	11

*"Agree" combines the answer categories of "agree" and "agree strongly" and "Disagree" combines "disagree" and "disagree strongly" were quite small. The exceptions were "It is better to use willpower to solve problems than it is to use tranquilizers (35 percent agreed strongly) and "Long-term use of tranquilizers may cause real physical harm to your body" (25 percent agreed strongly).

Source: Manheimer, D. et al., "Popular Attitudes and Beliefs About Tranquilizers," *American Journal of Psychiatry*, Vol. 130, p. 1246 (1973). Reprinted with permission.

TABLE 7.2. Percentage Condoning Drug Use for Anxiety and Depression under Various Conditions of Social Functioning (n = 2,241)

Condition	Drug for Anxiety	Drug for Depression
In work context		
1. To enhance normal functioning	13	8
2. To offset moderate deficit	55	38
3. To offset major deficit	64	50
In family context		
4. To enhance normal functioning	19	17
5. To offset moderate deficit	48	37
6. To offset major deficit	62	48

Source: Manheimer, D., et al., "Popular Attitudes and Beliefs About Tranquilizers," *American Journal of Psychiatry*, Vol 130, p. 1246 (1973). Reprinted with permission.

Results, shown in Table 7.2, indicate a willingness to condone either type of drug use to correct a significant deficit in function, but not to improve normal functioning. An interesting paradox was reported by the researchers, however. One-fifth of those condoning drug use in the case of moderate impairment would not do so in the more severe case. Comments from some respondents reflected the belief that severe mental problems require more physician intervention. There was also more support for use of the anxiety agent than the depression drug, probably, according to the researchers, because the description of the latter may have resulted in a mental linkage with "pep pill" use.

Yet another interesting insight into public attitudes is gained from comparisons between "general" attitudes and beliefs about tranquilizers and responses to condoning drug use. In effect, it was found that substantial proportions of respondents with generally negative attitudes toward the tranquilizers would still support their use in some of the situations described in the functioning questions. An intriguing finding was that "issues of morality, behavioral consequences, and efficacy are more influential in the decision to condone use than are beliefs about negative physical consequences." Clearly, these drugs carry some heavy social baggage.

Then Manheimer and colleagues took a clever and unusual step. How did the attitudes toward the drugs fit the respondents' larger value orientation? In an effort to find out, they constructed a "stoicism-traditionalism" index consisting of the following four items to which respondents could indicate "true" or "false":

Even if a person has troubles there is no reason why he cannot keep up a
cheerful front.
We should bear our troubles bravely and not complain.
There is something wrong with a person who is not willing to work hard.
I always follow the rule "business before pleasure."

Six other statements involving satisfaction with life were also used, with two
of them making up the remainder of the scale:*

I have always done my work to the best of my ability.
I have lived a moral and respectable life.

In a nutshell, the findings confirmed the pharmacological Calvinism
thesis. The higher the score on the stoicism-traditionalism index, the greater
the agreement that taking tranquilizers is a sign of weakness. There was
little variation on views concerning the physical risks.

The belief system was even more complex, however. Another statement used in the study was, "One of the main causes of mental illness is lack
of moral strength or will." About 40 percent agreed with that statement,
but those who did were more than twice as likely to view taking
tranquilizers as a "sign of weakness." Thus, "moral weakness causes
mental illness and taking tranquilizers to correct or ameliorate the condition
is further evidence of that weakness."

The conclusions of Manheimer and colleagues (1973) from their study
were as follows:

> There is considerable evidence that Americans believe in the efficacy of
> psychotherapeutic drugs but have doubts about the virtue of using
> them. . . . many people feel that the use of drugs that simply alter a mood
> or emotional state may mask symptoms or reduce motivation to change.
> Others feel that such drug use is clearly a moral or characterological
> issue. . . . Beliefs about psychotherapeutic drugs do seem to reflect a
> general moral stance—particularly concerning the values of strength and
> self-denial associated with the Protestant ethic. Consistent with such
> values is the finding that people are very unlikely to condone the use of a
> psychotherapeutic drug except in situations involving a real threat to
> important relationships or the ability to carry on important activities,
> such as work.

---

*Scoring is a bit complicated, but the range of the resulting overall scale was 0–6.

Those who had used the drugs were found to be more favorably disposed to them than those who had not, but even among the users there were real observations about such use. The research team found evidence of this conservatism in their utilization studies (see Chapter 4).

In the late 1960s, Gerald Klerman had coined the term "pharmacological Calvinism" in the context of a discussion of social atttiudes toward drug use. At the time, he noted poor documentation of public attitudes and beliefs about drugs, a situation that has improved only somewhat.

Klerman (1970) defined three drug ideologies:

1. That of the "Drug Hawks," who believe that nonmedical drug use is criminal, requiring strong, coercive legislation and law enforcement.
2. That of the "Moderates," who include many professional groups. Tobacco and alcohol are acceptable in moderation, but only a minority of moderates support legalization of marijuana.
3. That of the "Heads," who advocate freedom of drug use.

Klerman argued that the 1960s reaction to the drug-taking ideology was partly a result of the fact that the white middle class began to be affected, but also because of the influence of the protestant ethic.

In his view, components of the protestant ethic include the following:

1. Emphasis on individual achievement.
2. Belief that status, authority, and power arise from individual accomplishment.
3. View that gratification and rewards are to be earned by performance and valued for that reason rather than as ends in themselves.
4. Belief that logic, intellect, and rationality rather than intuition, revelation, and emotional experience are the path for Truth.
5. Belief that the Good Life comes from achievement and reason and that emotion and bodily satisfaction are to be disavowed.

Clearly, youthful LSD use, for example, flies in the face of these views. It is less clear, and Klerman does not so state in this paper, that use of minor tranquilizers can be lumped together with the more obvious types of drug abuse. Nevertheless, pharmacological Calvinism, as he defined it, exposes the view that "if a drug makes you feel good it must be bad. Indeed, if a drug makes you feel good, it's either somehow morally wrong, or you're going to pay for it with dependence, liver damage, chromosomal change, or some other form of secular theological retribution." (Klerman left out lung cancer, but the point is clear enough.*)

IMBALANCE OF USE BETWEEN WOMEN AND MEN

It is quite clear that women use and have used more minor tranquilizers, on the average, than men. It is not so clear what the reasons are, although many have been offered.

Hesbacher et al. (1975a) have both reviewd the literature and conducted research on the relationships among various social factors and the appearance of neurotic symptoms in family practice. From their research, it appears that "sex, race and social class correlate individually with the patient's reporting of emotional symptomatology." In regard to total symptomatology, it seems that race masks a true social class effect. In effect, it was found that there was an inverse relationship between social class and how "sick" the people were.

They noted the predictor effect of sex and conjectured that women may be socialized to report more psychoneurotic symptoms than men and that physicians may be socialized to "hear" more of the symptoms from female patients (similar to the Cooperstock model). They pointed out that such differences can be detected *only* after the patient has sought care, and therefore contribute little to the knowledge of etiology.

Finally, Hesbacher and colleagues were concerned about the possible inability of the primary physician to distinguish between legitimate and "labeled" (i.e., someone has told the patient he or she is crazy) symptomatology. To the extent that this concern is well founded, the physician may actually confirm the sick role in patients for whom it is appropriate.

Ruth Cooperstock is well known for her analysis of the special relationship between being female and the use of psychotropic drugs. In one report (1978a), she listed three models that have been used to account for differences in the illness experience of men and women. Model 1 simply states that it is culturally more acceptable for women to be and to report themselves as ill. Model 2 says that the sick role is more compatible with

---

*It is impossible to know what would have been the public's response to the minor tranquilizers had they not achieved prominence at the same time as the "drug culture" of the 1960s. Or was the latter merely a product of the development and use of the tranquilizers, as some will argue (i.e., sexual revolution = Pill or vice versa)? Would it have been possible for the minor tranquilizers to have been as successful without the success of the major tranquilizers that were first used on institutionalized patients?

women's other role responsibilities than with those of men. Model 3 argues that womens' assigned social roles are more stressful than those of men.

Certainly, the evidence indicates that women report more symptoms of neuroses and anxiety than do men and that they recieve many more prescriptions for minor tranquilizers. Many very serious observers charge that sex-role stereotyping functions in these statistics, asserting that male physicians have a general tendency to stereotype and devalue women relative to men, frequently misdiagnosing their presenting physical symptoms as psychogenic rather than organic in origin. It is not usually suggested that this tendency is malicious, rather that it is a natural outgrowth of medical school socialization and the influence of drug advertising (McCranie et al. 1978).

McCranie and colleagues (1978), in one of the few serious efforts to test the female stereotype charge experimentally, used clinical simulations to compare physicians' evaluations and clinical findings of male and female patients with identical presenting symptoms. No evidence of stereotyping was found. They concluded that if sex stereotyping does influence physician judgment, "it probably does so in concern with other patient characteristics and factors which need to be more clearly identified."

It may be that the stereotypes are kept alive at least in part by their critics. In any case, it is clear that there is a recurring stereotype of the beleaguered housewife, surrounded by small mountains of ironing and armies of children, "popping" Valium by the handful. As Brahen (1973) put it, "Many of these housewives flit from physician to physician to maintain a drug regimen no physician would prescribe." Unfortunately, data on this phenomenon are sparse, although Brahen presented figures on housewife drug abuse that were remarkably precise and equally remarkably free of any substantiation.

Nathanson (1980) used data from the National Health Interview Survey to explore the possible relationship between employment status and illness in women. She found employment to be positively associated with perceived health status, especially among women with fewer opportunities for self-esteem and social support outside of employment. Interestingly, sex differences in physician visits persisted even among employed women, leading Nathanson to suggest that "women are uniquely vulnerable to institutional pressures toward defining their problems in medical terms." [One comment seems appropriate here. Physicians have been criticized for drug treatment in women whose anxiety may be a result of low self-esteem. An alternative, of course, would be to alter the situation that causes this response. This is hardly possible for the physician, even through counseling. It should not be surprising (if not approvable) that the physician uses the means that are at hand—reduction of symptoms through prescribing minor tranquilizers.]

Mechanic (1978b) supported the institutionalized susceptibility to illness theory suggested by Nathanson. As he noted in his review of the data, women seem to report many more subjective symptoms than do men. Further, the excess of chronic illness among women seems to be, at least in part, a reflection of how they define and respond to illness and to their life situations.

Marcus and Seeman (1981) conducted research to assess the degree to which "fixed [i.e., inflexible] role obligations" contribute to male/female differences in reporting illness and disability. Their findings suggested that differences in sick-role behaviors are most likely when they conflict directly with fixed role obligations (e.g., when the individual must reduce normal activity).

Kessler and colleagues (1981) have also examined the sex differences in response to emotional disturbances. They found women to have a higher rate of emotional disturbance, but also, for the same symptom level, to be consistently more likely to seek psychiatric help. They hypothesized that their findings result from a greater likelihood among women to translate nonspecific feelings of distress into conscious recognition that they have an emotional problem than among men, and suggested that between 10 and 28 percent of the sex differential in treatment is due to this factor.

Noting the medical advertising that suggests use of antidepressants by mothers experiencing the "empty nest transition," Harkins (1978) studied that phenomenon. She concluded, from a study of 318 mothers, that (1) effects of empty nest transitions are slight and tend to disappear within two years and (2) physical well-being is not affected and psychological well-being is positively affected by the transition.

OTHER SOCIAL ISSUES

A frequent charge is that young people, seeing the consumption of minor tranquilizers and alcohol by their parents and other adults, are moved to experiment with drugs themselves. It is an appealing position both to young drug users and to adults opposed to drug use. For the former, it is a convenient excuse. For the latter, it provides a strong (and emotional) basis for argument against use. Mellinger (1971), however, formally studied the alleged relationship and found that young people (aged 18–29) were not emulating the over 30s, but rather "in this area of life as in many others . . . establishing new trends."

Mellinger's study, based on interview with 1,164 persons carefully selected in Contra Costa County, California, found women to be more likely than men to use tranquilizers. On the other hand, men were clearly heavier users of alcohol. Younger users were more likely to bypass the conventional medical channels of obtaining prescription drugs, less likely to use such drugs on a regular daily basis, and more likely to use stimulants than other classes of drugs.

What is the "meaning" of tranquilizers and their use?

Cooperstock and Lennard (1979) employed a "natural history" approach to assess the meaning of tranquilizer (benzodiazipine) use to 68 participants in group interviews and 24 authors of lengthy letters. Most were long-time users whose initial reason for use of the drug was a somatic problem in just over one-half of the cases. As the authors pointed out, however, the continuing use of the drugs is not explained by the biomedical (somatic) model of disease. Rather, it is clear that the majority continued to take the drugs because of a variety of role strains.

The use of a prescribed drug to cope with a social malady (role strain) raises a number of questions, as Cooperstock and Lennard noted. Some of their respondents ceased drug use "after making structural changes in their lives." Are such alternatives open to all members of society? The poor? The elderly? If not, are tranquilizers to be accepted as adequate solutions to social stresses?* These are clearly moral and ethical issues that transcend the bounds of the medical profession and demand social, not medical answers.

Helman (1981) used an anthropological approach to reach some very unusual conclusions about the symbolic meaning of the drugs themselves used over the long term. Helman classified long-term use of psychotropics as "tonic," "food," and "fuel." Those using the drugs as a tonic tended to use them more as a form of self-medication, to use them less frequently, and to be somewhat "antidrug." "Fuel" users saw the drug not as preventive against personality disintegration, but as a means of conforming to the expectations of significant others. Those who viewed the drugs as a kind of "food" tended to express least control over the use of the drug. Their ingestion occurred at fixed times with inflexible dosages, and they tended to be more "prodrug" in their attitudes.

Food, fuel, or tonic, Marks (1972) believes that, like the poor, some sort of chemical relief will be always with us.

> That humanity at large will ever be able to dispense with Artificial Paradises seems very unlikely. Most men and women lead lives at the worst so painful, at the best so monotonous, poor and limited that the urge to escape, the longing to transcend themselves if only for a few moments, is and has always been one of the principal appetites of the soul.

---

*For the poor, the answer is apparently "no," at least in states in which minor tranquilizers are excluded from the Medicaid formulary (see Chapter 9).

Even if not an "artificial paradise," it seems probable that escape will be sought. Whether the physician should be involved and at what point have been and will continue to be central issues in the consideration of the role of these drugs in our society. This is not a decision that has been addressed by the drug manufacturers. Nor is it appropriate to expect. The issue is a social one and it is the larger society that will have to resolve it.

A major and widely debated social issue remains the role of the physician, especially in the treatment of mental illness. A large philosophy of medicine symposium held in 1976 focused largely on this issue. One of the participants, philosophy professor Alan Donagan (1978), asked the question, "How much neurosis should we bear?" Donagan's question followed from two lines in a poem, "New Year Letter," by W. H. Auden:

> Give to each child that's in our care,
> As much neurosis as the child can bear.

Donagan's analysis suggested that Freudian theory might seem to argue, rather, that "as little [neurosis] as we can contrive" might be the answer to his question. He proceeded to argue that some neurosis is normal, perhaps beneficial, and that "everybody is at least incipiently neurotic."

Donagan pointed out that "we are more intimately identified with our minds than with our bodies," and that the vexations of neurosis may sometimes stimulate individuals to resolve their personal problems, thereby reaching a greater degree of self-knowledge. Such a viewpoint, however true, provides little aid to the physician, especially the general practitioner.

H. Tristran Engelhardt (1978), in his introduction to the symposium proceedings, provided several viewpoints relevant to the physician's dilemma: "If one takes seriously that being in the world is always physical, one must also accept that all mental activity has a physical reality." He further argued that physical conditions have mental components and vice versa, summarizing neatly the argument for prescribing tranquilizers in the presence, or even anticipation, of physical ailments. Evocative of arguments described elsewhere in this book, he stated:

> Attempts to draw clear lines between true diseases (i.e., somatic diseases) and problems of living (i.e., mental diseases) have not been successful. In fact, such distinctions would require some sort of Cartesian dichotomy between the body as a bearer of diseases, and the mind as a perpetrator of problems of living.

For the physician, these Cartesian considerations may be fascinating, but hardly practical guidelines for dealing with the anxious patient. As Engelhardt observed:

> No clear line can be drawn between the role the physician plays under the aegis of the mechanical medical model and the role he or she plays under this aegis of the mental illness model. The role of the physician is rather a broad and inclusive one, best described as that of a provider of remedies for complaints.

And it is that role, of course, which the physicians play when they provide minor tranquilizers for the complaint of anxiety, a practice targeted for criticism by many. What is the physician to do? Philosophy would seem to reply in the words of one of C. Northcote Parkinson's physicians, "Alas, we don't know."

For the physician—many dilemmas.

8

DOCTORS' DILEMMAS

> "The same society that demands the
> best of physicians is now creating the
> conditions that make it difficult for them
> to offer their best."
>
> Norman Cousins (1984)

In 1980, Dr. Louis Lasagna published a collection of "point/counter-point" papers under the broad title *Controversies in Therapeutics*. Dr. John Morgan drew the challenge of the position that perhaps our society is not overmedicated. The benzodiazepines were one class of drugs that he discussed in a cogent and pragmatic fashion:

> Everyone seems to know that we are an overmedicated society, and one
> imagines editors of publications small and large, common and arcane,
> swallowing benzodiazepines while rushing to meet a deadline with an
> article on the overmedicated society.

Lasagna's book exemplifies well the proposition that physicians face many dilemmas in their choice of drug therapy. Further, the use of the term "controversies" in the title illustrates the divergence of opinion that often exists. Among the controversial types of therapy were β-blockers, antacids, aspirin, opium derivatives, and, of course, benzodiazepines.

Morgan's chapter specifically addressed the issue of Valium use. He noted that Valium has an ample supply of both critics and defenders, and that, curiously, both sides tend to buttress their arguments with the same findings and data. Some of Morgan's comments offer an appropriate staging for our brief discussion of the dilemmas that the minor tranquilizers have brought to the prescribing physician.

One reason we stumble over questions of "appropriate" drug utility is our lack of understanding of the cultural context of drug use. We are asked to define a "proper" level of medication in society when we do not understand the social utility of powerful chemicals.

It is presumptuous—even preposterous—to define appropriateness solely from a clinical view.

Until we make more progress in defining the social utility of drugs and the social utility of health and well-being, it behooves us to be a bit more humble about appropriateness.

Diagnosis and conventional medical thought have essentially nothing to do with the usual use of benzodiazepines.

Morgan refers to a "somewhat tattered army of academics" caught between those who argue, forcefully, both sides of the "overmedicated" issue. Equally tattered, certainly, must be the practicing physician trying to make prescribing decisions while awaiting some resolution of the conflict between the political and medical leadership. The foregoing history surely demonstrates some of the physicians' dilemmas, which will be reviewed briefly here.

THE "DO SOMETHING" DILEMMA

In his book *Profession of Medicine*, sociologist Eliot Friedson (1970) argued for the activist orientation of the medical practitioner: "The aim of the practitioner is not knowledge but *action*. Successful action is preferred, but action with very little chance of success is to be preferred over no action at all." He further noted that sociologist Talcott Parsons had observed that activism is, in fact, a basic part of the American value system

Physicians, themselves action oriented, are thus faced with an "anxious" patient who also expects something to be done. Further, given the notoriety of the minor tranquilizers, the patient is likely to know that something can be done. On what basis can physicians withhold antianxiety therapy?

THE DEFINITION/DIAGNOSIS DILEMMAS

Although there are paper and pencil anxiety tests and clinical algorithms for diagnosis of clinical anxiety, these are relatively recent developments. Physicians have had no mental sphygmomanometer with which to measure mental pressure as with blood pressure. They do what they can, but rather well.

The detection of psychiatric illness is increasingly becoming the responsibility of nonpsychiatric physicians. As part of a large-scale epidemiological survey of psychiatric illness in a metropolitan area, primary care MDs and osteopaths were compared for their ability to detect psychiatric illness. Although neither group of physicians detected as much illness as patient self-assessments revealed, osteopaths detected significantly more psychiatric illness than MDs. When, however, physician and patient reports of illness were juxtaposed, to determine concordance, MDs and osteopaths showed similar degrees of overall accuracy. Osteopaths tended to detect more true positives, whereas MDs detected more true negatives. Different practice and social characteristics were not found to account for practice differences in physician rates of psychiatric illness detection. Osteopaths appeared to be performing at least as effectively as MDs in a first line of defense against mental illness (Hesbacher et al. 1975b).

A recurring medical problem is the difficulty in diagnosing and treating depression. While this may seem removed from the present subject, it is not, for depression is apparently often misdiagnosed and consequently treated as anxiety. Kline (1976) has called depression the "most misunderstood of all major diseases," advising that "any case of anxiety that does not respond to appropriate treatment within one to two months, should be reconsidered as possibly having an underlying depression. Many patients with such depression develop anxiety *secondarily* and do not respond to treatment until the primary depression is relieved."

The laboratory test, so helpful in other forms of illness, has not had much impact in this area. By 1980, however, some promise of progress had appeared. Gold et al. reported in 1981 that the use of a combination of the dexamethasone suppression test and the thyrotropin-releasing hormone test had high diagnostic value, although they warned against use "without regard for the entire clinical presentation or as a substitute for medical observation and judgment."

THE INFORMATION DILEMMA

How much of the information supplied by the drug manufacturers should physicians accept? How much should they believe? What are their alternatives?

Clearly, commercial information is biased, although the FDA has considerable authority to require a certain balance and to correct misleading messages. In any case, the information is palatable, convenient, and omnipresent. Further, the "scientific" information is often conflicting and sometimes (see Chapter 6) unscientific.

Although there are excellent textbooks devoted entirely to minor tranquilizers, it must be remembered that, for general practitioners at least, this is just one of scores of classes of drugs used daily. The AMA has released prescribing guidelines (reproduced below), but they appeared well into the "tranquilizer era" and well after many prescribing patterns were developed.

AMA Guidelines for
Administration or Prescribing
Psychoactive Drugs

1. Use barbiturates and other sedative hypnotics for relief of severe symptoms, but avoid them for minor complaints of distress or discomfort.
2. Attempt to diagnose and treat underlying disorders before relying on drugs of this class for symptomatic relief.
3. Assess susceptibility of the patient to drug abuse before prescribing barbiturates or any other psycho-active drugs. Weigh benefits against hazards.
4. Use dosages that will not lower sensory perception, responsiveness to the environment or alertness below safe levels.
5. Know how to administer barbiturates when clinically indicated for withdrawal in cases of drug dependence of the barbiturate type.
6. Using periodic checkups and family consultations, monitor possible development and dependence in patients who are on an extended sedative-hypnotic regimen.
7. Prescribe no greater quantity of a drug than is needed until the next checkup.
8. Warn patients to avoid possible adverse effects because of interaction with other drugs, including alcohol.
9. Counsel patients as to the proper use of medication—follow directions on the label, dispose of old medicine no longer needed, keep medicine out of reach of children, do not "share" prescription drugs with others.
10. Convey to patients through your own attitude and manner that drugs, no matter how helpful, are only one part of an overall plan of treatment and management.

Prepared by the AMA Committee on Alcoholism and Drug Dependence, and approved by the AMA Council on Mental Health and the AMA Department of Drugs.

THE MEDICALIZATION DILEMMA

In 1971, Lewis reported that nearly two-thirds of his (nonscientific) sample of physician respondents felt that other physicians were prescribing too many tranquilizers. He made clear through the example of a Valium advertisement his belief that a major reason for overprescribing was the "medicalization of human problems," noting that "once daily living is defined as disease, how logical it is for us to attempt to treat that disease."

Again, if one looks to Freidson's exposition on medicine, one finds an explanation, if not an excuse, for the medicalization of human problems. As he observes (and supports by argument), "The medical profession has first claim to jurisdiction over the label of illness and anything to which it may be attached, irrespective of its capacity to deal with it effectively." In fact, people come to physicians because there is anxiety in their lives. By the simple act of seeking medical assistance, the patient has medicalized the problem. Of course, by treating the patient, the physician confirms that this medicalization was appropriate. If the drug works, even if only briefly, the actions of both patient and physician are reinforced, and the drugs have worked—criticism of the effectiveness of the benzodiazepines, at least, has been rare.

One may argue (and many do) that the drugs do not "cure" the anxiety and do not eliminate the cause. True enough, but the same can be said of antihypertensive medication, antiarthritics, even aspirin. Should the patient be denied relief of mental discomfort when it is caused by problems of daily living?

Unless and until society is provided with an acceptable alternative to the physician in dealing with their personal problems, as long as they continue to seek relief from this source, it is unrealistic to expect the physician to turn them away because they have a problem with which he or she should not deal.

Society has medicalized human problems, it appears. Medicine has, perhaps, been an accessory, and the pharmaceutical industry, certainly, has provided both with the means. To expect either of the latter parties to do, or have done, otherwise bespeaks a considerable naiveté.

Freidson (1970) pointed out that "while medicine is hardly independent of the society in which it exists, by becoming a vehicle for society's values it came to play a major role in the forming and shaping of the social meanings imbued with such a role." He argued that physicians became "moral entrepreneurs," seeing "mental illness" where the layperson sees "nervousness" or "problems." Yet, that same layperson has come to the physician for help. If the physician eschews treatment (with drugs), the patient is likely to be disappointed (the activism value), and the physician becomes equally a moral entrepreneur, saying, in effect, "You were wrong to come to me. Pull yourself together and get your life in order." However correct that judgment may be, the personal burden on the physician can be enormous.

Primum non nocere, however! It is all very well for the physician to provide relief, but what about the attendant harms of addiction and habituation?

THE DILEMMA OF ADDICTION

It is clear that some minor tranquilizers may be addicting for some people, and habituating for even more. Physicians have an equally clear obligation to avoid such adverse effects in their patients. Again, however, it took a comparatively long period of time to demonstrate these dangers scientifically. And indeed there is still controversy (Marks 1972).

There are controls, perhaps belatedly established (see Chapter 9), designed to limit the abuse potential of these legitimate drugs. It should be pointed out, however, that some of the burden for misuse must be borne by others than the prescribing physician. With or without appropriate caution by that physician, refill prescriptions have been a major factor in the utilization pattern of the minor tranquilizers. The utilization statistics following the "controlling" of these drugs show a substantial decline in refills, indicating at least partial responsibility on the part of the patient and the dispensing pharmacist.

Is there a "Doctor Feelgood" extant in medicine? Certainly there must be, but there is scant evidence that he is ubiquitous. On the other hand, refill restrictions may not be the only answer.

In Great Britain, there are no refill prescriptions in the same sense as in the United States. The patient must return to the surgery, ostensibly see the physician, and receive a "repeat" prescription. In fact, this system, which would seem to offer a great opportunity to monitor patient therapy, does not always work so smoothly. Dennis (1979) studied 1,000 repeat prescriptions from three genral practitioners who did not see the patient when the prescription was issued. He found that one of ten patients who were receiving repeat prescriptions had been doing so for more than ten years. (The study included hypnotic and other drugs besides minor tranquilizers, although the latter made up 66 percent of all the prescriptions.)

Physicians seeking guidance have, again, been hard to put to find it. Ayd (1970) reached the following conclusions with regard to the abuse of minor tranquilizers:

1. The potential for abuse does exist.
2. The proportion of real abusers is so small as to be almost incalculable.
3. The abuse arises, not from some inherent property of the drugs, but rather from psychopathology in the user.
4. There is no evidence of a serious problem to society resulting from the low rate of abuse.

McNair (1973) reviewed some 20 years of research on the effects of antianxiety drugs on human performance and found them sorely lacking:

> Almost two decades of laissez-faire research in the area have yielded no adequate, systematic data base for meaningful inferences. About all one can safely and tritely conclude is that all these drugs affect performance under some conditions. There simply is no reasonable basis for generalizing about either the specific or the comparative effects of these drugs. Surely this deplorable net result of undirected and misdirected science and pseudoscience suggests that some routine should be established to provide a comparable data base for evaluating the effects on performance of any antianxiety drug marketed for administration to humans.

Maletzky and Klotter (1976) reviewed some 27 studies from the 1960s concerning diazepam. None of them, they concluded, included sufficient controls to warrant dismissing the question of addiction. Based on their review of research as well as their own studies, they asked, "There is not reason to doubt diazepam's efficacy in reducing levels of anxiety . . . but at what price?"

CONTINUING DILEMMAS

Dr. Frank Ayd (1970) has observed,

> The history of twentieth century psychiatry makes an exciting narrative of the evolution of psychodynamic and physical methods of treatment; of therapeutic nihilism yielding to a spirit of expectant optimism; of a struggle against prejudice, inertia and indifference; of the blossoming of multidisciplinary scientific interest in mental illness; of an unprecedented availability of money and manpower for psychiatric research; and of remarkable strides forward in the conquest of diseases of the mind.

He further noted that "tranquilizers and antidepressants now available have made it possible for all physicians, not just psychiatrists, to treat emotionally and mentally disturbed patients—something previously not

TABLE 8.1. Substitutes for Treatment with Psychotropics

If no tranquilizers were available . . .	Frequency of Mentions (n = 657) (%)
Longer medical consultations would be needed.	75.3
The patient would visit the doctor more frequently.	72.1
Psychotherapy would be required.	62.4
Patient would need a period in a sanitorium.	52.1
Patient could turn to alcohol.	50.7
Patient would require so much attention in the practice that treatment of other patients could suffer.	46.9
Patient would use preparations not recommended by doctor to treat organic complaints.	44.0
Patient would need to be hospitalized.	38.7
Patient would use addictive drugs.	36.5
Patient would have to be treated with medicaments that could be used to commit suicide.	34.4
Patient would have to undergo organic therapy.	28.9
Patient would have to be treated with preparations affecting the organism more seriously.	24.2
Patient would be in constant need of care and attention.	20.1
Patient would have to be sent to institution or home.	18.1
Patient could require operation.	5.6

Source: From Contest: *Psychopharmaka—Arztebefragung*, Volume of statistics, Frankfurt on the Main (1974), quoted in Marks (1972).

possible." Of course, there was no guarantee that they would do it well, and Ayd observed, "The sad truth is that not enough doctors have mastered the art of psychopharmacotherapy, and that this accounts for the divergent therapeutic results and complications reported by different therapists."

Marks (1972), in his monograph of benzodiazepine dependence, quoted a German study that showed physician responses to a question concerning the consequences of the unavailability of tranquilizers. (No distinction was made between major and minor.) As the results, shown in Table 8.1, indicate, the consequences might be serious.

Few objective observers have suggested elimination of the minor tranquilizers. *Stopping Valium* (Bargmann et al. 1982, p. 17), as harsh a critique as one is likely to encounter, says, "We do not advocate banning Valium." Just the same, the criticism continues, and it encompasses, by either direct accusation or implication, physicians, pharmacists, patients as individuals, the pharmaceutical industry, and society at large. Each of these groups must ultimately deal with the issues, but the prescribing physician is certainly a central character.

The physician's frustration and its interaction with social values are well illustrated by a recent study of patients who were negatively stereotyped by physicians (Najman et al. 1982). This study, which found remarkably consistent results among more than 2,400 Australian and American physicians, showed "patients with minor medical disorders" to be consistently negatively stereotyped (along with patients and substance abusers). The researchers' attempts to explain their findings included three approaches, which are illuminating to this discussion of doctors' dilemmas.

The first explanatory approach describes middle-class sanctioning of deviance from traditional values of "hard work, an emphasis on achievement, an avoidance of over-indulgence, a stress on self-discipline and cleanliness and a willingness to defer gratification." The second approach would explain the negative stereotyping as resulting from the failure of the patient with minor mental conditions to fulfill the "sick role." The third explanation is situational, involving the physician: "The difficulties and uncertainties associated with the presenting symptoms produce a realistic negative reaction by the doctor."

We should not be surprised, then, if, faced with these dilemmas, "even physicians who use these drugs frequently seem to suffer from some guilt and join in the criticism" (Morgan 1980).

CULTURAL LAG AND THE MINOR TRANQUILIZERS

A number of years ago, Paul Stolley (1971) discussed the cultural lag in health care. As he put it:

> Sociologists have long observed that changes do not occur in a coordinated way even in closely related parts of our culture. Technological advances commonly outstrip the ability of society to adapt to and utilize these advances. This delay is called "cultural lag" by sociologists.

As noted in Chapter 1, we believe the minor tranquilizers are an example of such a cultural lag.

Regardless of the company provided our misery by other technological advances, the fact remains that we now have the benefit of a quarter-century of experience with medications having important social significance. Certainly, there are other drugs in the making that will offer equal problems and opportunities. Perhaps we have learned something. As comedian Lily Tomlin says, "Maybe if we listened, history wouldn't keep repeating itself."

In any case, the formal mechanisms that society uses to deal with its problems have not been unaware of the minor tranquilizers.

9

TRANSIENT SITUATIONAL DISTURBANCES: THE REGULATORY ENVIRONMENT

> "If a law is not absolutely necessary, then it is absolutely necessary that there not be a law."
>
> Lord Acton

With the possible exception of narcotics, it is unlikely that any class of drugs has received as much legislative and regulatory attention as have the minor tranquilizers. In this chapter, we review in considerable detail the proceedings of congressional hearings that, directly or indirectly, sought to define an appropriate role for these drugs. The activities of the FDA as well as other regulatory agencies are also surveyed. Throughout, the picture is one of evolutionary development influenced by politics, scientific progress, money, and (not always informed) opinion.

CONGRESSIONAL HEARINGS

Former Commissioner of Food and Drugs Alexander M. Schmidt (1978) has provided a very familiar view of the FDA and the politico-regulatory process:

> The following scenario is being repeated all too often in Washington: a scientist, somewhere in the world, in a speech, paper, or press release, presents his or her conclusion that a particular drug is a carcinogen, a teratogen, or whatever. The press picks this up, recognzies the sensational news value of the story, checks only whether the scientist actually released it, and then reports the story widely. A congressional staff member, sensing the story's sensational news value to his or her

employer, arranges a hearing into the matter. At the hearing carefully selected witnesses testify to the overuse and misuse of the drug, which FDA is called upon to explain. FDA is urged strongly to do something about the problem; there is another round of sensational press reports; and eventually, regulations are proposed.

Of course, the psychotropic drugs were special. As Aden (1978) has observed,

> The empirical value of treatment with psychopharmacologic agents may not serve in and of itself to prevent further unwarranted legislative or judicial intrusions upon its domain, for it is clear that the brain and the central nervous system, different from the rest of the body, are viewed as something special—the essence of existence!

For these and other reasons, the minor tranquilizers have frequently been the subject of or part of a number of congressional hearings.

The Blatnik Hearings*

House hearings were conducted early in the tranquilizer era under the direction of John Blatnik (Minnesota). His Subcommittee on Legal and Marketing Affairs of the House Committee on Government Operations met for four days in February 1958 to study "False and Misleading Advertising of Prescription Tranquilizing Drugs." The stated purpose was an "inquiry into the activities of the Federal Trade Commission in the control of false and deceptive advertising of medical preparations."

The first witness was Dr. Nathan Kline, then director of research at Rockland State Hospital in New York. Kline cited the salutory effects of the major tranquilizers on psychiatric inpatients and reported that, to his knowledge, not a single case of addiction to psychopharmaceuticals had been reported "although habit formation and dependence are as common as might be expected."

In his discussion of advertising, Kline stated, "[The manufacturers] have to earn a living, and, if promotion keeps them in business, then hurrah for promotion, since this is the only way they will be able to contribute to the research effort." Nevertheless, Kline noted some potential problems in promotion, among them the quotation of research results out of context, the "leaking" of scientific information to the popular press, and over-enthusiasm. He concluded, however, "that the excesses which were

---

*References to congressional hearings may be found in the Bibliography under the name of the chairperson.

indulged in, unquestionably, by some of the pharmaceutical houses have virtually disappeared."

Representatives of the AMA appeared before the subcommittee and received a thorough grilling. Some of the testimony was rather strange, e.g., this exchange between Dr. Leo Bartemeier, chairperson of the AMA Council on Mental Health, and Congressman Meader of Michigan:

> Mr. Meader. Well, now, your position is chairman of the American Medical Association council on mental health?
> Dr. Bartemeier. That is right.
> Mr. Meader. If anyone in the American Medical Association were to know of misrepresentations and information sent by pharmaceutical houses to the medical profession with respect to these tranquilizer drugs, would not you be the one to know about it?
> Dr. Bartemeier. I do not think I would; not necessarily.
> Mr. Meader. Well, are you aware—
> Dr. Bartemeier. The function, the main function of the Council on Mental Health, sir, of the American Medical Association, is to be of assistance to physicians in the application of the basic principles of psychiatry in the practice of medicine. This has not anything to do with drugs, you see.
> Mr. Meader. But drugs are a part of your activity, are they not?
> Dr. Bartemeier. A minor part.
> Mr. Meader. In health?
> Dr. Bartemeier. I would say a secondary part. You see, we are more concerned with what is mental; we are more concerned with those deviations from health which we ordinarily speak of as mental; that is, as psychic. We are far less concerned in our particular field with the physical aspects of medicine.

Congressman Meader tried, unsuccessfully, to wring from Dr. Bartemeier some criticism of drug advertising:

> Mr. Meader. In your profession or in the medical profession beyond psychiatrists, have you heard of any complaints that the literature sent by the pharmaceutical houses has contained misrepresentations or misleading information?
> Dr. Bartemeier. No; I have not. I have heard doctors say that they did not get the results that they expected, but I could not say that that was due to misrepresentation on the part of the manufacturers of the drugs.

Dr. Ian Stevenson, professor of neurology and psychiatry at the University of Virginia, was more critical of advertising, noting in his testimony three important offenses:

1. The presentation of data in advertising brochures gives an appearance of high scientific quality without the data in fact possessing this.
2. The advertising of the drug manufacturers frequently fails to give proper emphasis to complications and side effects of the drugs. Drugs that can in fact have quite serious complications may be presented as possessing only minor hazards, when careful studies have shown this not to be so.
3. The advertising of the drugs can include a serious oversimplification of mental illness and its cure, leading the unwary physician and patient to believe that the answer has already been found.

Dr. Albert Holland, then medical director of the FDA, was asked to clarify the respective roles of the Federal Trade Commission (FTC) and the FDA regarding the regulation of drug advertising in medical journals. He struggled with the answer inasmuch as the FDA's jurisdiction, at that time, was limited to labeling, and journal advertising could hardly be viewed as labeling, or could it?

Dr. Holland. This would be an exceptional instance, Mr. Plapinger, and one which we have never really encountered, or certainly an action on the part of the Food and Drug Administration which we have to date, to my knowledge, never employed. I think it would be possible, however, with some of the interpretations of court decisions in the past to take a journal advertising piece which appeared in a journal and which was in a physician's office and somewhere else in his office either a free sample that had been furnished him or perhaps even a package of material which he had purchased for dispensing to his patients, and I think under unusual circumstances, and I am not suggesting that we do this, one could establish in the purely technical sense that this is labeling which accompanies the product in that it is written, printed or graphic material.

Mr. Plapinger. I see. Is it proper to imply from your statement that you feel that the primary jurisdiction in this field, at least, is with the FTC, rather than the FDA?

Dr. Holland. Yes.

Mr. Meader. Might I ask a question on that for clarification, to clarify a further point? But if you didn't find the drug in the physician's office, if he only had the medical journal and he simply wrote out a prescription and the drug was in the drugstore, never in his office, then you would have no authority to call that labeling; is that correct?

Dr. Holland. I think that is right with respect to that physician in that particular office, but there are 150,000 of them and sooner or later—

Mr. Meader. You will find a drug and a magazine together.

In August 1958, the subcommittee submitted its final report. It noted the problems of the FTC with regard to drug advertising.

FTC member Sigurd Anderson could recall

> no instances where the medical profession or any member thereof has complained that a drug advertisement disseminated exclusively to the profession contained a false representation of a material fact or that a *drug* did not contain a truthful disclose of its formula.

He conceded that the commission need not wait for an outside complaint but could—and does in other fields—initiate action of its own motion. Anderson referred to FTC manpower difficulties. The commission, he said,

> has only two doctors and I assure you that they are stacked up way beyond any load they can carry in other areas where we are conducting our investigations. Perhaps if we had doctors to examine as to the claim made in this type of advertising, we could do something, but at the present time I assure you we haven't.

After some comment, the subcommittee reached the following conclusions and recommendations.

1. The FTC has not discharged its statutory responsibilities to halt or prevent deception in the advertising of ethical tranquilizing drugs.
2. The Commission should institute trade practice conference procedures without delay with a view to effecting codes of fair advertising practices for ethical pharmaceutical firms.
3. Consideration should be given by the appropriate legislative committees of the Congress to determine whether statutory changes are required for more effective enforcement action in the field of false and misleading advertising.

Such consideration was, of course, subsequently given—at great length.

The Kefauver Hearings

Senator Estes Kefauver formally began his long and often controversial investigation of the drug industry with hearings on July 9, 1957. Testimony before his Subcommittee on Antitrust and Monopoly of the Senate Committee on the Judiciary was ultimately to span 16,000 pages and fill more than 26 volumes. The hearings would also lead, by a curious turn of events, away from Kefauver's initial target, the types of pricing and competition in the industry, and toward a major restructuring of the FDA and expansion of its powers with regard to drug approval and promotion. The Kefauver investigations have been chronicled by a number of authors, so we will limit our attention to their concern for the minor tranquilizers.

In some ways, at least in the present context, the most interesting portions of the hearings were those that focused on the "father of Miltown," Dr. F. M. Berger, and his relationship with the Carter Company, the parent firm of Wallace Laboratories.

Henry Hoyt, president of Carter, presented the lead testimony. He noted that the firm had purchased Dr. Berger's interest in Miltown, the company's "first successful ethical product." He also pointed out that some 40 competing tranquilizers had appeared since the introduction of Miltown in 1955 and added that Wallace was perhaps the only major drug company without a detail staff.

Hoyt described the price determination of Miltown as a process of surveying the prices of competing products and then setting a price "in line with the competition." There had been no increase in price in the four years since the product's introduction. Hoyt noted:

> A survey of the use of Miltown shows that the average dose is three tablets a day. the price to the patient is 10.6 cents a tablet, about the price of a cup of coffee or a candy bar. The average dose of three tablets a day, or a total cost of 31.8 cents a day, is comparable to the price of a pack of cigarettes or a gallon of gasoline. Of the 10.6 cents per tablet the patient pays, I have estimated Carter's profit to be about 1.2 cents per tablet.

Also described were Carter's license policies—a very important subject since they did not then manufacture their own meprobamate.

> In the United States, Carter reserves to itself the control of manufacture of the meprobamate powder. Licenses are given the right to manufacture tablets from our powder and to sell them.
>
> Carter is concerned that meprobamate powder be manufactured in accordance with rigid quality standards. The powder is difficult to manufacture. Therefore, we prefer to have it made under our control and supervision, and to assay the finished powder ourselves. Accordingly Carter has the product made by five manufacturers of its own selection to whom it has imparted its "know-how." We can terminate these relationships at any time if we are not entirely satisfied with the quality of production.
>
> Licenses have been granted to a number of other companies to market meprobamate in combination with other useful drugs, but we have done this only when there was good experimental and clinical evidence of therapeutic value.

Dr. Berger's own testimony focused on remarks made earlier in the hearings by psychiatrists Fritz Freyhan and Heinz Lehmann. He took strong exception to their views and method of presenting them.

> As a physician, I question the wisdom of discussing in a public forum the relative advantages or disadvantages of particular drugs. The efficacy of important drugs can well be minimized, or even completely destroyed, by statements which could affect the patient's confidence in the drug or in his physician. Such statements could lead to discontinuance of treatment against the best available medical advice.

Berger questioned the validity of published studies that suggested that meprobamate might be addicting, and stated that there was "no evidence indicating any abuse of tranquilizers." He also defended drug advertising:

> The purpose of the advertisement is to remind the busy practitioner of the availability of the drug and its general attributes and not to contain a full presentation as in the reference manual. We have confidence in their intelligence and sense of responsibility to know they will prescribe the drug, not on the basis of a one-page ad, but on the basis of substantial information in the medical journals and their own experience in the use of the drug, as well as the experience of their colleagues.

Senator Kefauver, however, noted that Miltown advertisements up to that point in time had never mentioned any side effects for the drug, and further that some ads explicitly stated that it had no side effects. Berger did not respond.

Presumably because the focus of the hearings was on drug costs, the committee explored in detail Dr. Berger's compensation.

> Mr. Dixon. According to this report, Dr. Berger's income for the fiscal year ending March 31, 1957, was as follows:
> His salary was $35,500. He recieved executive compensation in the amount of $18,000 and income from Carter's purchase of meprobamate patent in the amount of $113,000. According to information that we have from the Securities and Exchange Commission for the year 1958, Dr. Berger received $295,755. I am not clear whether that is total, whether that includes salary and executive compensation and his royalty, or whether it is just royalty compensation.
> That is 1958. Now we understand in 1959 you paid him $344,000. In addition to that amount in 1959, he received salary?
> Mr. Hoyt. That is correct.
> Senator Kefauver. What was his salary in 1959?

Dr. Berger. $80,000.

Senator Kefauver. He made $344,000 in royalties plus $80,000 in salary?

My. Hoyt. I would like to point out though, if I may interrupt, that this payment to Dr. Berger is mostly in payment for a patent which he developed, and I have had similar arrangements with other scientists who have worked with us.

I believe that when a scientist develops anything, he should share in the fruits of his developments and this I think, this idea of not paying scientists for what they develop I think is all wrong.

So I don't think you should consider this compensation to Dr. Berger. It is payment. He sold something which he had the right to.

Senator Kefauver. That's right. We want to encourage scientists. But I must observe that $295,000 in 1958, plus his salary and $344,000 in 1959, that is getting way up there for a little company, isn't it? You are doing pretty well.

Kefauver concluded his examination of the Carter Company by stating: "I think your prices to the American druggists are way too high." He was concerned about the compensation levels of the executives and observed:

It wouldn't make an awful lot of difference to me if this concerned some luxury item that only very wealthy people could buy and sometimes maybe foolish people who want to spend their money; I don't much care how much they have to pay or how much the company makes. But here we are dealing with something different, something in which there is a great public interest. We are dealing with something that people must have, drugs—poor people, middle income people, as well as wealthy people. They have no alternative. So there is a different responsibility. I think you have a responsibility to all the people.

What might happen? Kefauver would have to vote "no" to any government control of prices, but he was afraid that the American public might bring strong pressures to bear on Congress.

Meanwhile, Berger's ire had been aroused by comments such as these from Dr. Fritz Lehmann, a psychiatrist from Montreal. Lehmann began by making the important distinction between the major and minor tranquilizers—with a bit of editorializing.

There are two classes of tranquilizing drugs, and this is somewhat obscured by the nebulous term, "tranquilizer," which is not a scientific one, but a popular one which now has become the label also in scientific journals. One is the class of what one might call the major or "big gun" tranquilizers, which are really effective in major mental diseases and have produced almost revolutionary changes in mental hospitals because of their therapeutic impact.

The other class of tranquilizers, the one that most of the advertising literature is about, are usually simply glorified sedatives of the older class. They are advertised for anxiety states, tension states, and are not effective in the major mental diseases for patients in mental hospitals, for instance. And one will always have to ask distinctly what kind of tranquilizer one is referring to: class 1, which has proven its effectiveness in mental hospital patients, or class 2, which may or may not be effective against anxiety and where the effect is mainly of a symptomatic nature.

Lehmann was also concerned about the charges of overuse, addiction, and habituation.

If the minor tranquilizers are abused, prescribed too much, taken too much, then there is a danger of addiction. Certainly as regards one of them, Meprobamate, Miltown, Equanil and sold under various other trade names, it has been proven that large doses over a long period of time, over several weeks, may produce addiction just as barbiturates. Also, there always is the danger of psychological dependence. In other words, somebody who is used to taking pills at the slightest upset he feels will finally become incapable of tolerating any kind of stress and will become dependent on a pill at the slightest bit of tension that he feels, and that may stifle his spontaneity, his creativeness, his independence. So there are dangers, psychological and physical dangers, with the minor tranquilizers.

In his written, prepared testimony, Lehmann singled out meprobamate.

Of these less important tranquilizers, one Meprobamate (Miltown, Equanil) has for years assumed the leading role. It has become popularized in cartoons, TV quips, through a tremendous advertising campaign, and has convinced people of its merits by giving them temporary, short-lasting relief of unpleasant tension states without producing any other unpleasant side-effects. There is, in my mind, no doubt that the abuse of the minor tranquilizers and of Meprobamate in particular is tremendous.

Criticism of advertising during the hearings focused primarily on two issues, whether Miltown was habit forming or addicting and the degree to which warnings concerning side effects were included (or omitted) from the ads. It was noted that Carter had failed to supply ads for study, necessitating their retrieval from the Blatnik Committee.

Lehmann noted that where previous ads had explicitly stated "non-addictive," then current ads used the phrase "well suited for prolonged therapy." Prior discussions had singled out one advertisement that conveyed the impression that the drug had no side effects at all.

The hearings provided interesting insights into the intercorporate negotiating process as well. Documents obtained by the committee illustrated the process by which Carter negotiated worldwide licensing agreements as well as agreements to combine Miltown with the patented drugs of other firms.

Combination Products and Licensing Agreements

Smith Kline and French.   Smith Kline and French was already a leader in the psychotropic drug field, having marketed chlorpromazine under the trademark Thorazine through a licence with Rhone-Poulenc. In June 1955, Berger indicated by internal memo that Smith Kline and French was interested in selling meprobamate as a "superior mephenesin" Nothing came of this, however, although the possibility of combining Miltown with both Thorazine and with Dexedrine was also explored.

Schering.   Negotiations with Schering were more fruitful, however. In November 1955, Schering expressed an interest in combining meprobamate with their steriod products Meticorten and Meticortelone. Three days later, Carter expressed interest as well. Possible indications for the combination were related to muscle problems.

Nearly a year later, an internal memo from Berger to Hoyt showed continued interest by Schering in a Miltown-Meticorten combination. There was some haste to market the product "before the Atarax-Meticorten combination gains a foothold."

The Schering correspondent (Dr. "Skeeter" Lee) had stated:

1. Only 14 days will be needed for the preparation of the New Drug Application (!).
2. Schering has no objection for Merck-Sharp and Dohme to sell the combination as well.
3. Schering will let us have a phenothiazine derivative allegedly 15 times better than chlorpromazine.

A week later, Berger had cooled to the idea of a Schering connection, recommending instead an agreement with Merck. His reasons:

1. Merck was anxious to enter the prednisone market; Schering anxious only not to lose it.
2. Merck seemed likely to achieve quick action on a new drug application.

3. Schering was already marketing several Meticorten combinations.
4. Schering would not grant Carter a license on prednisone, "showing a lack of good faith."

Licensing Agreements

Carter reached a number of international licensing agreements as well as domestic ones.

American Home Products. American Home Products was licensed to "use and sell, but not to manufacture" meprobamate, which they did, as Equanil, through their subsidiary, Wyeth. In June 1957, a further agreement between the two firms resulted in the combination of Wyeth's conjugated estrogen product, Premarin, and Miltown.

Lederle. Under a 1957 agreement, Lederle Laboratories, a division of American Cyanamid, was licensed as a major international distributor of Miltown. Further agreements resulted in the marketing by both firms of a combination of Miltown and Pathilon (Carter, Milpath; Lederle, Pathibamate).

In fact, although the Kefauver Hearings provided interesting insights into the developing minor tranquilizers industry, these drugs were not the main focus of these proceedings.

The Humphrey Hearings

Then Senatory Hubert Humphrey, himself a pharmacist, was responsible for a series of Hearings on Interagency Coordination in Drug Research and Regulation. Some of these proceedings touched on the minor tranquilizers. Humphrey noted the earlier work of Congressman Blatnik when he introduced his first witness, Dr. Fritz Freyhan, who had appeared earlier with Senator Kefauver.

Freyhan was now in charge of clinical studies at the National Institutes of Health. He was still concerned about "overuse, if not abuse" of the minor tranquilizers. "In a way," he stated, "the drugs became everybody's business before their usefulness had been sufficiently determined."

Among the issues raised by Freyhan during this testimony was a full-page advertisement for Librium that had appeared in the March 15, 1963, issue of *Time* magazine. The ads appeared in issues of *Time* that had been sent only to physician subscribers. Nevertheless, Freyhan was concerned about two things. First, he felt the content of the ad was misleading, suggesting that "nervous breakdown, cardiac neurosis, and peptic ulcer" might "be avoided by the timely use of this drug." There was, according to

Freyhan, "no shred of evidence to lend substance to such claims." In addition, he was concerned that the magazine, with the ad intact, might find its way to the physicians' waiting rooms and therefore patients.

The publisher of *Time* responded by describing the measures undertaken to alert the doctors to remove the ads and defending the accuracy of the advertising message itself. One month later, the House of Delegates of the Medical Society of the State of New York passed a resolution disapproving of such advertising. Editorials in medical journals followed. *GP*, the journal of the American Academy of General Practice, stated, "It is incredibly clear that many of the 'physician only' pages will not be removed." Such ads, said *GP*, "should not appear in *Time, Playboy, Humpty Dumpty* or *Popular Mechanics.*" The *New England Journal of Medicine* took a somewhat different view: "The public is entitled to all the knowledge of health and disease that can reasonably be made available to it." Thus, although medical journals might not like the lay competition, they saw no reason why physicians should worry if the information in *Time* reached the consumer.

The committee spent considerable time on the issue of habituation, and requested and received from the FDA the chronology that is reproduced here to illustrate the tortuous path of regulatory action even in these comparatively early days.

1. On 12/16/54 the first New Drug Application for a drug containing meprobamate was filed. It was filed by Wallace Laboratories, New Brunswick, N.J.
2. The application was allowed to become effective on 4/28/55.
3. The next New Drug Application for a meprobamate product was for Equanil submitted by Wyeth Laboratories, Inc., Philadelphia, Pa. It was made effective on 7/26/66.
4. On 1/28/57 Dr. Weilerstein of the Bureau of Medicine, assigned to San Francisco, received a "Clinical Bulletin" from Wallace Laboratories declaring: "Habituation does not follow the use of Miltown. Withdrawal symptoms have been completely absent in this study and in two previous studies with *** neuropsychiatric patients *** because of its complete lack of toxicity and side effects in moderate dosage. Miltown is an ideal drug for repeated use, as in premenstrual tension."
5. On 1/31/57 Dr. Barbara Moulton wrote to Wallace Laboratories stating that the above described mailing piece had just come to her attention, and in view of the fact that habituation, withdrawal symptoms and other toxic effects have been reported with Miltown, the entire tone of this bulletin was misleading.
6. On 2/6/57 Wallace Laboratories, Inc., wrote to the Food and

Drug Administration agreeing to change the mailing pieces and to submit a revised brochure in the near future.

7. On 2/8/57 Wallace Laboratories submitted to the Food and Drug Administration a revised brochure. About the same time, Wyeth Laboratories submitted a revised brochure for their product, which was considered satisfactory.

8. In a telephone conservation of 5/1/57, and in a letter of 5/6/57, Division of New Drugs informed Wallace Laboratories that its brochure should be revised along the lines of the Wyeth brochure.

9. On 5/8/57, Wallace Laboratories submitted a further revised brochure which contained under "Side Effects" the following:

"Lemere has raised the question of possible habit formation, particularly in those patients prone to excessive self-medication and dependence on other agents who are most often affected and withdrawal symptoms have occurred in these. Lemere states that 'Meprobamate is not addictive in respect to any increase in tolerance. On the contrary, one of the big advantages of this drug is that with continued medication decreasing amounts are usually needed to produce the same effect'.

"Careful supervision of dose and amounts prescribed for patients with a known tendency or potential for taking excessive quantities of drugs is advised. Where excessive dosage has continued for weeks or months, dosage should be gradually reduced rather than abruptly stopped, since the withdrawal of a 'crutch' may precipitate an anxiety reaction of greater proportions than that for which the drug was prescribed."

10. On 7/3/57 Dr. R. G. Smith wrote to Wallace Laboratories making their supplemental application covering this brochure effective.

11. During the months following this action, reports came to the attention of FDA that drug withdrawal reactions in patients who had received larger than recommended doses for considerable periods of time were occurring, and on 1/28/58, a conference was held with Doctors A. H. Holland, R. G. Smith, and E. R. Jolly of the FDA and Dr. F. M. Berger of Wallace Laboratories and Dr. G. E. Farrar of Wyeth Laboratories.

12. At this conference it was agreed that the following steps should be taken:

(a) In the brochure for Miltown and Equanil under the heading "Side Effects" the following paragraph would be included:

"Careful supervision of dose and amounts prescribed for

patients is advised; especially with those patients with a known propensity for taking excessive quantities of drugs. Excessive and prolonged use in susceptible persons, for example, alcoholics, former addicts, and other severe psychoneurotics, has been reported to result in dependence on the drug. Where excessive dosage has continued for weeks and months, dosage should be reduced gradually rather than abruptly stopped since sudden withdrawal may precipitate withdrawal reactions. These have, in some cases, taken the form of epileptiform seizure."

(b) The first page of the brochure would bear a similar or identical statement set in prominent type under the heading "Important."

(c) Rough draft of the changes in the brochure would be submitted within a few days and final printed brochures as soon as available.

(d) To insure wide distribution of this information, the brochure would be used as a package insert and also a general mailing of it to all physicians would be made. It was also agreed that any other major mailing piece of meprobamate would also include the substance of the quoted statement in (a) above.

(e) The following statement would be deleted as not in accord with the fact:

"Meprobamate is not addictive in respect to any increase in tolerance. On the contrary, one of the big advantages of this drug is that with continued medication decreasing amounts are usually needed to produce the same effect."

13. Draft copy of the revised brochure incorporating the changes agreed upon was received from Wallace Laboratories on 2/25/58.

14. On 3/4/58, Dr. Jolly of New Drugs Division wrote to Wallace Laboratories making their supplemental New Drug Application for the revised brochure effective.

15. Wyeth's brochure was treated in like fashion and the supplemental NDA for a similar brochure was also permitted to become effective.

In the exhibits included in the committee record were early reports from the *Medical Letter*. The very first issue of *The Medical Letter* (January 1, 1959) had focused on meprobamate. The review was harsh: "The widely held belief that meprobamate has virtues in relieving anxiety and tension that are unique or different from those of barbiturates does not appear to be justified by available evidence." Further, "the available evidence also leaves no doubt that addiction can be induced with meprobamate." The editors made the interesting observation that "it may be that the intensive promotion of meprobamate and the publicity it has received in the lay press give it special virtues as a placebo." Nearly two years later (October 28, 1960), the *Medical Letter* found meprobamate inferior to barbiturates (and more costly).

The Dingell Committee

Congressman John Dingell's Subcommittee on Regulatory Agencies began hearings in April 1967 to investigate Small Business Problems in the Drug Industry. Minor tranquilizers figured in these proceedings primarily because they were large-volume sellers and therefore a focus of competition between chain and independent pharmacies.

Harold Goldfeder, a pharmacist from Riverdale, Maryland, told the committee that "many large outlets are taking what we call 'hot' items, the most popular items and selling them at reduced prices." One of the "hot" items was Miltown.

> One of the chains in the area sent out a bulletin to their pharmacists and they are getting $6 a hundred on a prescription from the consumer, and yet you see that the lowest price, if an independent drugstore operator purchased this from a wholesaler, the lowest price he could get it for would be $6.12.

In January 1968, the committee heard testimony from Roche delivered by Irwin Lerner, then general manager of the Pharmaceutical Division. Again, the committee was interested primarily in pricing and distribution policies, but other issues were raised.

Committee Counsel Potvin noted that some pharmacists had complained about product "proliferation." One of the products that might be an example of such "proliferation" was Roche's Libritabs. Mr. Lerner saw the introduction of this dosage form in a different light.

> Mr. Lerner. Libritabs is in essence a tablet form of the Librium capsule. It is virtually indistinguishable in therapeutic effect on a milligram-for-milligram basis. Libritabs was developed in response to the medical profession's request for a tablet form of Librium, which had been available for some time in the capsules to which I refer. Now, why? Some patients have difficulty in swallowing capsules, and they require that the medicine be administered in tablet form. To prepare a launch of a product like Libritabs required 5 years of processing for a new drug application

which covered extensive clinical investigation of the product's efficacy, its effectiveness and its safety. It covered the years approximately between 1961 and 1966.

In addition to this, to the fact that the medical profession did need this and that subsequent sales have fully justified its existence in the marketplace on the basis of its therapeutic merit, no pharmacy by virtue of our liberal return goods policy needs to keep Libritabs in stock so that except for direct accounts which by virtue of our introductory shipment policies have agreed to keep it in stock for 6 months to give us a chance to create the demand to get it moving through, they can return it for virtually any reason and receive full or partial credit. So we don't consider this—we consider this rather an example of implementing our policy of introducing only those drugs which offer something by way of safety, effectiveness, or practicality and not a deliberate policy of proliferation.

[No one apparently thought to point out that physicians sometimes wish to give patients the appearance of changing medication without actually doing so. Libritabs, different in name and appearance from Librium capsules, made this possible. An older Roche product, Alurate (amobarbital), which was introduced as a red liquid, was later joined by Alurate Verdum, a green liquid containing the same ingredients.]

After Senator Ester Kefauver's 26-volume hearings proceedings were published, as well as the 7-volume work of Senator Humphrey's hearings, Langer, writing in *Science* in 1965, reported a diminished congressional interest in drug matters: "Industry executives are anticipating their most restful season in years." Langer noted interest in drugs by Abraham Ribicoff (later secretary of health, education, and welfare), Philip Hart, and L. H. Fountain, but the name of Senator Gaylord Nelson did not surface.

The Nelson Hearings

About the same time of the Dingell Hearings in the House, Senator Gaylord Nelson (Wisconsin) opened hearings of his own on Competitive Problems in the Drug Industry. The Nelson Hearings were to have a much longer run, rivaling Kefauver in length of time and volume. These hearings, which began in May 1967, continued until 1979, filling 34 volumes and more than 17,000 pages of testimony and exhibits. The Nelson Hearings were also notable for their attraction to *Washington Post* writer Morton Mintz, whose book, *The Therapeutic Nightmare*, had its genesis in the earlier Kefauver era. Through much of the hearings, Mintz and Nelson enjoyed a relationship (at least in print) not unlike that of Howard Cosell and Muhammed Ali in the sports world.

Four days of testimony and one volume of the Nelson Hearings were devoted specifically to psychotropic drugs, but these drugs were also discussed in other testimony. Indeed, in the second session (June 1967) of the subcommittee (Part 1), Boston physician Richard Burack, who had just published *Handbook on Prescription Drugs*, singled out Wallace Laboratories as one company with objectionable advertising. He testified:

> In June 1964, Wallace Laboratories advertised a product called Pree MT which contained both meprobamate—Wallace's brand name: Miltown—a hydrochlorothiazide—which has three different brand names. The Government charged that the advertisements falsely claimed: "Contraindications: None known." Wallace Laboratories pleaded *nolo contendere*, thus avoiding a trial and *attendant publicity*.

In August 1967, Dr. James Goddard, then commissioner of the FDA, testified concerning progress in implementing the provisions of the 1962 Drug Amendments. He submitted in evidence "Dear Doctor" letters that the FDA had required of Wallace and Roche to correct prior promotional messages. (They are reproduced as Figures 9.1 and 9.2, respectively.)

In March 1969 (Part 2), the subcommittee received written testimony from Dr. Dale Console, former medical director of E. R. Squibb and Company. Console singled out two examples (one of which is included here) "to demonstrate the kind of advertising that apparently meets the new FDA requirements."

> [Figure 9.3] is in extremely poor taste not only because the woman depicted in the photograph can be suffering from anything from simple exhaustion, to anemia, through chronic schizophrenia, and on to any chronic debilitating disease, but also because it is only slightly, if at all, removed from the crass television commercials that say she has "tired blood" and needs Geritol, or those that say she has the "blahs" and needs AlkaSeltzer. She needs careful diagnostic work-up and not a prescription for Valium t.i.d. or q.i.d. The advertisement is a total composition deliberately intended to convey the impression that the "always weary" (a diagnostic category unknown to me) can be treated by writing a prescription for Valium.

> A question that is frequently asked, and it is invariably asked in a tone that conveys amazement and total disbelief is: "Do doctors actually prescribe on the basis of advertising?" This device was used frequently in the Kefauver Hearings and most witnesses avoided the question since an affirmative answer left one open to the accusation that he was questioning the intelligence and integrity of his colleagues.

Dr. Console also supplied a copy of testimony that he had given the Kefauver Committee nearly 10 years earlier. It included these comments.

Wallace Pharmaceuticals
Division of Carter-Wallace Inc.
Cranbury, NJ

Dear Doctor:

At the request of the Food and Drug Administration, we are calling your attention to one of our recent advertisements captioned, "The published clinical studies indicate: 3 of 4 non-psychotic depressions respond to 'Deprol.'" The FDA considers that this advertising may have been misleading.

In the advertisement, we listed 21 studies comprising the total published 'Deprol' literature containing data on non-psychotic depressions. While the ad does not reflect the fact, data from these studies were excluded in whole or in part if—

(a) the diagnosis was not entirely clear;
(b) the recommended maximum dose of 6 'Deprol' tablets per day was exceeded;
(c) other psychotropic drugs or electroshock were counted as therapy.

Moderate, marked, excellent, and complete responses were counted as favorable, while mild, fair, slight, and no responses were counted as unfavorable.

Using the above criteria, the final number of patients included was 323 selected from ten of the 21 listed studies. Nine of the ten studies were uncontrolled, and most patients in the ten studies concomitantly recieved informal or structured psychotherapy. The reported therapeutic results (ranging from 0% in a study with two non-psychotic depressed patients, through 64% in a study with 53 such patients, to 90% in two studies with 38 and 41 such patients respectively) also include, to an undetermined degree, placebo responses and spontaneous remissions known to occur in the therapy of neurotic depression.

The factors noted above represent problems that exist in working with any literature and are present in some 'Miltown' advertisements carrying the theme "one of a series." In order to avoid any misunderstanding, we have discontinued the use of these 'Miltown' advertisements as well as the described 'Deprol' advertisement.

Sincerely,

WALLACE PHARMACEUTICALS

FIGURE 9.1 Wallace Letter

Roche Laboratories
Division of Hoffmann-La Roche, Inc.
Nutley, NJ

Dear Doctor:

At the request of the Food and Drug Administration, we are extending the "brief summary" of prescribing information for Librium[R] (chlordiazepoxide HCT) which appears in medical journal advertisements by adding several phases and items from the unchanged official package circular.

The revised "brief summary" for medical journals is attached, indicating by capitalization the requested added material. Prescribing information in all Librium (chlordiazepoxide HCT) package circulars, direct mail information and brochures is complete and requires no change. The safety and effectiveness of the product are not in question.

In addition, in future medical journal advertisements for Librium (chlordiazepoxide HCt) in geriatric patients, we are amplifying statements which have appeared concerning possible side effects and initial dosage:

The statement that "Side effects in most instance are mild in degree and readily reversible with reduction of dosage," will be extended by the observations made in our package circular which point out that drowsiness, ataxia and confusion have been reported in some patients, particularly the elderly and debilitated, occasionally at lower dosage ranges, and that in a few instances syncope has been reported.

Whereas in geriatrics, the usual daily dosage is 5 mg. two to four times daily, the initial dosage in elderly and debilitated patients should be limited to 10 mg. or less per day, adjusting as needed and tolerated.

We hope the additional detail in medical journal advertising clarifies the use of the product in accordance with the enclosed package circular.

Sincerely,

Robert E. Dixon, M.D.
Director, Professional Services

FIGURE 9.2 Roche Letter

175

BRIEF SUMMARY OF PRESCRIBING INFORMATION FOR LIBRIUM
(Chlordiazepoxide HCL)

(NOTE.—This revised "brief summary" for use in future medical journal advertising contains additional phrases and items (printed in capital letters) from the official package circular which remains unchanged.)

Before prescribing, please consult complete product information, a summary of which follows:

Contraindications.—Patients with known hypersensitivity to the drug. Warning.—Caution patients about possible combined effects with alcohol and other CNS depressants. AS WITH ALL CNS-ACTING DRUGS, CAUTION PATIENTS against hazardous occupations requiring complete mental alertness (E.G., OPERATING MACHINERY, DRIVING). THOUGH PHYSICAL AND PSYCHOLOGICAL DEPENDENCE HAVE RARELY BEEN REPORTED ON RECOMMENDED DOSES, USE CAUTION IN ADMINISTERING TO ADDICTION PRONE INDIVIDUALS OR THOSE WHO MIGHT INCREASE DOSAGE: WITHDRAWAL SYMPTOMS (including convulsions), following discontinuation of the drug and similar to those seen with barbiturates, have been reported. Use of any drug in pregnancy, lactation, or in women of childbearing age requires that its potential benefits be weighed against its possible hazards. Precautions.—In the eldery and debilitated, and in children over SIX, limit to smallest effective dosage (INITIALLY 10 MG OR LESS PER DAY) TO PRECLUSE ATAXIA OR OVERSEDATION, increasing gradually as needed and tolerated. NOT RECOMMENDED IN CHILDREN UNDER SIX, THOUGHT GENERALLY NOT RECOMMENDED, IF COMBINATION THERAPY WITH INDIVIDUAL PHARMACOLOGIC EFFECTS, PARTICULARLY IN USE OF POTENTIATING DRUGS SUCH AS MAO INHIBITORS AND PHENOTRIAZINES. Observe usual precautions in presence of impaired renal or hepatic function. Paradoxial reactions (E.G., EXCITEMENT, STIMULATION, AND ACUTE RAGE) have been reported in psychiatric patients and hyperactive aggressive children. Employ usual precautions in treatment of anxiety states with evidence of impending depression; suicidal tendencies MAY BE PRESENT AND PROTECTIVE MEASURES NECESSARY. Variable effects on blood coagulation have been reported very rarely in patients receiving the drug and oral anticoagulants; causal relationship has not been established clinically. Adverse reactions.—Drowsiness, ataxia and confusion may occur, especially in the elderly and debilitated. These are reversible in most instances by proper dosage adjustment, but are also occasionally observed at the lower dosage ranges. IN A FEW INSTANCES, syncope HAS BEEN REPORTED. Also encountered are isolated instances of skin eruptions, edema, minor menstrual irregularities, nausea and all infrequent and generally controlled with dosage reductions; changes in EEG patterns (low-voltage fast activity) may appear during and after treatment; blood dyscrasias (including agranulocytosis), jaundice and hepatic dysfunction HAVE BEEN REPORTED occasionally, making periodic blood counts and liver-function tests advisable during protected therapy.

FIGURE 9.2 (cont.)

Usual daily dosage.—Individualize for maximum beneficial effects. Oral—Adults: Mild and moderate anxiety and tension, 5 or 10 mg. t.i.d. or q.i.d.; severe states, 20–25 mg. t.i.d. or q.i.d. Geriatric patients: 5 mg. b.i.d. to q.i.d. (SEE PRE-CAUTIONS.) Supplied.—Capsules, 5 mg., 10 mg., and 25 mg.—bottles of 50.

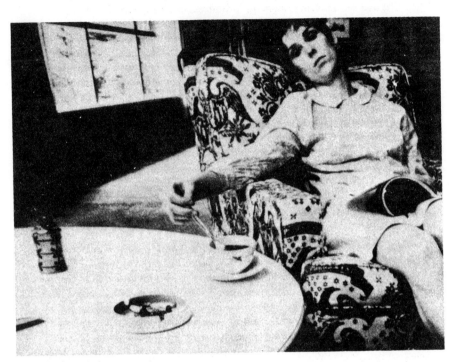

Psychic support for the "always weary"

When psychic tension is the reason for chronic fatigue, Valium (diazepam) can help provide the right kind of support. That's because, in proper dosage Valium calms the tense, tired patient while seldom dulling the senses or interfering with function.

In this way, the patient may be better

FIGURE 9.3

177

A better approach is one which is used frequently in the promotion of so called tranquilizers, but with minor variations spreads to many other drugs. Either in the course of legitimate investigation or in the search for a new promotion device it is found that a drug which is claimed to be effective in relieving anxiety, produces, in rats, specific objectively measurable changes in a particular area of the brain. Now this is an interesting truly scientific finding but in the present state of our knowledge its significance is unimportant since it is both intriguing and impressive. It is presented in an advertisement or a brochure complete with accurate anatomical illustrations of the brain beautifully executed in vivid colors. This is coupled with the claim that the drug relieves anxiety. The usual response of the average practitioner who is not, and is not expected to be, an expert in neuro-physiology is to associate the two and to assume that they support each other.

In May of the same year, the subcommittee discussed drug combinations. Dr. John Adriani, then of Charity Hospital in New Orleans, supported labeling prescriptions with the generic name of the drug involved. Meprobamate was one of the examples used.

Here is an example with which I am familiar. A patient went to one physician and was treated by that physician for some time. He did not think he was getting any better. So someone else said, "Why don't you go to see my doctor?" He had been given Equanil by this first doctor. The other doctor looked at him and said to himself, this fellow is on the "neurotic side," and I will give him Miltown. So this patient threw away his Equanil and bought Miltown. Miltown is the same thing as Equanil. If meprobamate had been on the label and the patient had seen that label, he would have said "he gave me the same thing the other doctor did." And he would have said, "maybe there is something wrong with me 'upstairs.'" And he would have known that he got the same medicine.

Nelson opened the meeting on psychotropic drugs with a prepared statement:

When Aldous Huxley wrote his fantasy concept of the world of the future in the new classic "Brave New World," he created an uncomfortable, emotionless culture of escapism dependent upon tiny tablets of tranquility called soma.

It was chillingly disconcerting to read Huxley's book like figures frantically hiding from reality. It was comforting, however, that the book was after all only science fiction. But in the nearly 40 years since Huxley created his classic the fiction began to read like reality. It became a prophetic insight into the kind of society we seem to be moving toward today.

In our complex society we have our soma to escape the frustrations. We find our psychotropic drugs to escape in barbiturates and tranquilizers. Over the past few years, if we can believe only a small part of what has been written, Americans have been insulating themselves from the pressures of modern life by using tranquilizing drugs in rapidly increasing numbers.

Our problem is that we don't really know very much about the tranquilizing drugs or what they are doing to us as individuals and to our society as a whole. These hearings will be seeking answers to what many thoughtful people believe to be vitally important questions. To my knowledge, no one has gathered the best information available in one place on psychotropic drugs. We hope to begin that competition today.

Dr. Stanley Yolles, the first witness and then director of the NIMH, had concerns as well.

To what extent would Western culture be altered by widespread use of tranquilizers? Would Yankee initiative disappear? Is the chemical deadening of anxiety harmful? To what extent are the Peyote cultures different because of the use of mescal, or Central American tribes unique because of their hallucinatory mushrooms?

I would add here, when it comes to a seduction, it takes a seductor and a seductee. And I feel that myself and my colleagues—or it seems to be evident from the sales statistics—are so easily seduced by the clever advertisement.

Senator Nelson subsequently responded, agreeing that the physicians must share some blame:

There has to be a better way of advertising drugs. Only I think sometimes the blame is too one sided. Something must be done also about physicians' critical ability to understand what kind of information they are depending on. Somehow I feel the blame tends to be somewhat one sidedly on the ad without enough criticism directed at the physician who, for lack of training on the one hand, and for reasons of simplicity and gullibility on the other hand, depends for his prescribing information, to a large extent, on clever advertising.

Another critic of psychotropic drug advertising was Dr. Richard Pillard, assistant professor of psychiatry at Boston University. Pillard supplied a number of examples including an ad for Valium, which, according to his testimony, omitted important scientific background information. He was also critical of Vistaril ads showing an anxious child, noting that "this appears in general medical journals although even specialists in child psychiatry seldom use tranquilizers and then only for limited and specific indications." Among Pillard's recommendations were (1) discontinuation of advertising in medical journals; (2) discontinuation of free samples; and (3) a serious reconsideration of promotional policy by the drug industry.

Nelson's next witness, Dr. Daniel X. Freedman, was professor of psychiatry at the University of Chicago. He was more positive in his attitudes toward the minor tranquilizers.

> The so-called minor tranquilizers—the sedative antianxiety agents which have their greatest use in general medical practice—have probably enhanced the flexibility and efficiency through which the physician can offer effective treatment in a variety of medical contexts.
> So I am not willing to throw out the sedative antianxiety drugs as a banality. The fact that you and I both know that society can exist without them doesn't mean that either of us have assessed the cost in human suffering.

The final witness was anthropologist Margaret Mead, whose testimony was remarkable. Some of it is reproduced below:

> We also have, as a part of our tradition, what is called the Puritan ethic, in which we democratically attempted to spread the practices of abstinence, sobriety and the postponement of all gratifications, hopefully to heaven or at least until a man got rich, throughout the entire population. The Puritan tradition, which has been a very important one in our country, was remarkably successful in promoting economic development and the Industrial Revolution, also includes a very strong bias against any chemical of any sort which alters mood, makes life seem less difficult than it is, puts one to sleep when one is kept awake by worries, relaxes one when one should stay tense, and so forth.
>
> There is a general emphasis in this country upon finding external solutions to all problems; if you don't like where you are living move somewhere else; if you haven't got any land make it; if you have the wrong shaped nose get it fixed; if you have too big a nose and to small a chin take a piece of your nose and put it on your chin and don't complain that you are going to have to sing in the choir or as a spinster all your life. Right straight through our history we have adopted a policy that invention, techology, ingenuity, resources ought to be available to deal with anything that we want to have dealt with.
> These three attitudes occur, in different mixtures in different constituencies, in different parts of the country and in different individuals, including the advertisers who advertise for the pharmaceutical industry and the detail men and the physicians who receive their ministrations. The practice desire to fix things come into conflict with a belief that some measure of pain is part of man's lot in the world. If you carry that far enough you use no analgesics of any sort in childbirth because pain is what man was born to and woman was condemned to and she should continue to bear the pain.

Senator Nelson was concerned that Dr. Mead might be suggesting that it would be healthy for people to avoid all stresses. She responded,

No; I think it is very unhealthy for them to avoid facing stresses of the order of death or even moving and separating from their friends. But I do believe it is worthwhile to avoid the stress that comes when the plumbing breaks down and both cars are broken and you can't find your husband to telephone him, and the child in nursery school, three children in nursery school, you were going to pick up 15 miles somewhere else, if a pill will permit you not to burst into tears under these circumstances but go next door and borrow another car, I think it is a good idea and I don't think we should confuse the inevitable stresses of the complexity of modern life with the great moments in man's existence which he has to face up to.

I think that a good deal of the testimony against psychotropic drugs, and particularly anxiety reducing drugs, is of this sort and confuses the issues.

The Fountain Hearings

In December 1970, the Senate Committee on Government Operations (the "parent" of the Blatnik Subcommittee) submitted its report on Regulation of Prescription Drug Advertising. The report noted significant improvement in the quality of drug advertising following the enactment of the 1962 advertising amendments to the Food, Drug, and Cosmetic Act, but noted that serious problems remained.

Within a few months, Congressman L. H. Fountain (North Carolina) convened hearings by his Subcommittee on Intergovernmental Relations to Study the Safety and Effectiveness of New Drugs, subtitled Advertising and Promotion of Prescription Drugs. His first witness was Dr. Charles Edwards, then commissioner of the FDA, and the Serentil ad was still an issue (Figure 9.4).

> Mr. Fountain. I recall from the committee report that an earlier misleading ad for Serentil appeared late last year. And FDA requested that Sandoz Pharmaceuticals stop advertising the drug as a treatment for alcoholism on September 24, 1970. Is that correct?
>
> Dr. Edwards. That is correct.
>
> Mr. Fountain. In that instance the manufacturer complied with FDA's request to discontinue the ad. But FDA did not request a corrective ad or any other remedial measure because it had approved the false labeling claim that Serentil is effective in the treatment of alcoholism. As indicated in our report, FDA believed this approval deprived it of "an impressive legal basis for requesting additional remedial measures such as a corrective ad or a 'Dear Doctor' letter."
>
> This was the basis for our recommendation 6 that FDA review all existing prescription drug labeling for accuracy, for completeness, and for clarity.
>
> So it appears that the manufacturer ran a second ad on Serentil in 1970 which FDA also found to be misleading. I have here a copy of that ad taken from Medical World News December 11, 1970 which contains in the large type caption "For the Anxiety That Comes From not Fitting

FIGURE 9.4

In" and also told how it was misleading.

Dr. Edwards, I wonder if you would tell us briefly what you found wrong with the original advertising and why you believed the corrective ad was necessary in this case?

Dr. Edwards. If I might, Mr. Chairman, I would like to have Dr. Simmons (Director, Bureau of Drugs) answer that question.

Mr. Fountain. Dr. Simmons, all right.

Dr. Simmons. Mr. Chairman, the Serentil campaign that you just showed was corrected because in our opinion this drug, a phenothiazine, is inappropriate for use for the problems of everyday living. We therefore called in the firm, pointed that out to them, and requested a corrective ad. That ad was run in the same journals in which the original ad had run (Figure 9.5).

As a further point of interest, in the same edition of one of the journals in which that corrective ad was run, an editorial appeared which in some respects supported our action by saying that these drugs probably were being overpromoted for the indicated uses.

Mr. Fountain. Then in the corrective ad, you requested that they state wherein the advertising was misleading. I might read the substitute language for a good portion of the new ad which says in a boxed legend: "Published to correct a previous advertisement which the Food and Drug Administration considered misleading. Serentil"—and then it gives the content of the tablets and so forth.

"The Food and Drug Administration has requested that we bring to your attention a recent journal advertisement for Serentil (mesoridazine) which featured the headline 'For the Anxiety That Comes From Not Fitting In.'

"The FDA considers the advertisement misleading in several respects. For example: the FDA states that the principal theme of the ad suggests unapproved uses of Serentil for relatively minor or everyday anxiety situations encountered often in the normal course of living. The fact is that Serentil, a phenothiazine drug, is limited in its use to certain disease states (see opposite page for indications) in which the risk of phenothiazine therapy is justified in the opinion of the physician.

"We have taken steps to withdraw the advertisement in question."

Corrective advertising was continued to be used by the FDA.

Drug Abuse Control Amendment Hearings

In early 1970, Congressman Paul Rogers convened hearings on the above amendments that were aimed primarily at further efforts to control drug abuse. The minor tranquilizers were discussed, however.

Dr. Frank Ayd was one witness who was concerned about some of the potential adverse effects of the proposed amendments. Ayd had "yet to see an abuser of a major or minor tranquilizer or an antidepressant." He noted that the Drug Abuse Control Amendments of 1965 had been aimed at amphetamines and barbiturates, but that in 1966 the FDA had proposed

PUBLISHED TO CORRECT A PREVIOUS ADVERTISEMENT WHICH THE FOOD AND DRUG ADMINISTRATION CONSIDERED MISLEADING

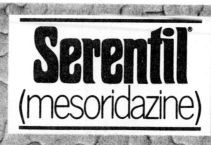

Serentil®
(mesoridazine)

TABLETS 10 MG., 25 MG., 50 MG., AND 100 MG.
MESORIDAZINE (AS THE BESYLATE)

THE FOOD AND DRUG ADMINISTRATION HAS REQUESTED THAT WE BRING TO YOUR ATTENTION A RECENT JOURNAL ADVERTISEMENT FOR SERENTIL (MESORIDAZINE) WHICH FEATURED THE HEADLINE "FOR THE ANXIETY THAT COMES FROM NOT FITTING IN."

THE FDA CONSIDERS THE ADVERTISEMENT MISLEADING IN SEVERAL RESPECTS. FOR EXAMPLE:

THE FDA STATES THAT THE PRINCIPAL THEME OF THE AD SUGGESTS UNAPPROVED USES OF SERENTIL FOR RELATIVELY MINOR OR EVERYDAY ANXIETY SITUATIONS ENCOUNTERED OFTEN IN THE NORMAL COURSE OF LIVING. THE FACT IS THAT SERENTIL, A PHENOTHIAZINE DRUG, IS LIMITED IN ITS USE TO CERTAIN DISEASE STATES (SEE OPPOSITE PAGE FOR INDICATIONS) IN WHICH THE RISK OF PHENOTHIAZINE THERAPY IS JUSTI-FIED IN THE OPINION OF THE PHYSICIAN.

WE HAVE TAKEN STEPS TO WITHDRAW THE ADVERTISEMENT IN QUESTION.

FIGURE 9.5

adding minor tranquilizers to the list of controlled substances because of their depressant effect on the central nervous system. A trial examiner had upheld this contention, but Ayd strongly disagreed.

If there were abuse, Ayd believed that a solution lay not in controlling the drugs, but in controlling their use.

> Even if chlordiazepoxide, diazepam, and meprobamate are put on the drug abuse control list, there will be abusers of these compounds until physicians: 1) exercise caution in prescribing these compounds for patients with a history of alcohol or drug abuse and for patients with character disorders, and 2) restrict the amount ordered, limit refills, and regularly monitor their patients carefully. Potential abusers of medicine can be detected in most instances if the physician thoroughly examines the patient, noting his behavior in the office, and takes the time to determine how the individual has used drugs previously and his drinking habits. Although lifelong inadequate personalities may manifest symptoms for which minor tranquilizers may be indicated they usually are not suitable candidates for these compounds.
>
> Clearly one way of reducing the risk of drug abuse is for the medical profession to train physicians who are honest and efficient in action, who are aware of the value of human life and the hazards to which they expose patients when they prescribe drugs, and who by perpetual vigilance and a persistent renewal of moral sensibilities are men who first do no harm. Such physicians are not created by legislative fiat.

Roche President V. D. Mattia, not surprisingly, was also opposed to controls on the minor tranquilizers, noting, among other things,

> If this Committee determines that minor tranquilizers should be subject to control, the legislation should provide a separate schedule with appropriate penalties for those drugs because of their safety, extensive medical use and their extremely low likelihood of abuse.

In explaining his position, Mattia stated:

> We recommend that a separate schedule be included in the bill for the minor tranquilizers and the long-acting barbiturates, such as phenobarbital. Clearly, these drugs must be separated in the schedules from the dangerous and widely abused, short-acting barbiturates and the amphetamines.
>
> This new schedule, interposed between Schedules III and IV of the Senate bill would:
>
> Have the same regulatory controls as those imposed on the drugs presently in Schedule III. For example, the same record-keeping and prescription limitations would be applied.
>
> Be distinguished by a different label symbol for the drugs it covered.

Make first offense violations a misdemeanor rather than a felony. This would reflect the minimal hazards involved in the misuse of these drugs and essentially parallel the sanctions applicable to drugs having a lesser potential for abuse, such as those regulated under Schedule IV of the Administration proposal.

This proposal for a schedule for minor tranquilizers separate from amphetamines and short-acting barbiturates makes good sense—scientifically, medically and legally.

Mattia buttressed his arguments with statistics on abuse levels of various substances and submitted letters from 35 police and regulatory officials stating that there was "virtually no illegal trafficking in Librium and Valium."

The Nelson Hearings on Advertising of Proprietary Medicines

In addition to his hearings on Competitive Problems in the Drug Industry, Senatory Gaylord Nelson also examined the Advertising of Non-Prescription drugs. During two sessions (in July and September 1971), his Subcommittee on Monopoly focused on the "mood drugs," and although officially aimed at nonprescription products, testimony did touch on the prescription minor tranquilizers.

An early witness was Dr. Charles Edwards, then commissioner of the FDA, who quoted Richard Nixon:

We have created in America a culture of drugs. We have produced an environment in which people come naturally to expect that they can take a pill for every problem—that they can find satisfaction and health and happiness in a handful of tablets or a few grains of powder.

How did this happen? Commission Edwards believed there were several reasons:

1. The increasing complexities and stresses of modern society.
2. The postwar discovery of chemicals that allegedly help the average person cope with these stresses and frustrations.
3. The tremendous wave of advertising over the media, especially television, creating an environment in which consumers feel that reaching for a pill, tablet, or capsule is a panacea for all of their ills.

Edwards was especially concerned about the advertising of prescription "mood drugs."

The manufacturers of prescription psychotherapeutic drugs are stretching the uses and the intent of the medications beyond their proven medical benefits.

The drugs are actually intended for patients suffering from anxiety and tension. These are psychiatric conditions which require careful diagnosis and management. They do not include the ordinary frustrations of daily living.

These comments and some advertising examples caught Senator Nelson's attention:

May I interrupt, Doctor? Isn't there a very fundamental distinction between prescribing a drug to help the patient manage a serious problem of depression and tension and prescribing a drug to help the patient meet the ordinary—as you put it—frustrations of daily living? In other words, isn't the difference between the two that one is, or may be, a medical problem and the other is one of the ordinary frustrations and tensions of daily living and not really a medical problem?

Dr. Edwards. That is exactly correct, Senator. I certainly wouldn't want any of my testimony misconstrued to the extent that we are trying to downgrade the role of the psychotropic drugs in the treatment of true mental illness. They have played a very important role but as you have indicated there is a real difference between the frustrations of daily living and true mental illness.

An advertisement for Librium came in for special attention.

Senator Nelson. What proof of efficacy is there for some of these prescription drugs under the statutory definition? For example, let us take the ad for Librium, the official name of which is chlordiazepoxide HCL. Here is a picture of a college girl carrying her books. At the top it says, "A whole new world of anxiety," and it says, "The new college student may be afflicted by a sense of lost identity in a strange environment. Today's changing morality and the possible consequences of her 'new freedom' may provoke acute feelings of insecurity. She may be excessively concerned over competition, both male and female, for top grades. Unrealistic parental expectations may further increase emotional tension. Her newly stimulated intellectual curiosity"—get this—"may make her more sensitive to an apprehension about unstable national and world conditions. Exposure to new friends and other influences may force her to reevaluate herself and her goals. Take Librium."

Then there is a page of warnings, precautions and so forth, which is not very conspicuous.

Now, what proof, what controlled clinical trials have been filed with the FDA to demonstrate that this drug is efficacious for treating these conditions?

Dr. Edwards. Well, we have none. I think it is important to point out that when these drugs were approved by the Food and Drug Administration these particular symptoms that you indicated, anxiety, tension, neurosis, and so forth, were part of a medical condition, a medical disorder. They were not approved for treating an everyday situation or ordinary life problem. What has happened is the advertisers, the promoters of these drugs, have taken these symptoms out of context and applied them to the day-to-day situations that we are all confronted with. As a result they have developed this totally misleading advertising.

This original approval of these drugs by the Food and Drug Administration was legitimate. We were thinking of these drugs in terms of medical conditions and not for use in ordinary life situations.

Senator Nelson. So, in other words, what you are saying is that when the drug company filed the New Drug Application and filed whatever proof of efficacy that is required—

Dr. Edwards. That is right.

Senator Nelson (continuing). The controlled clinical trials were for medical conditions only?

Dr. Edwards. That is exactly correct.

Senator Nelson. What would be defined as a medical situation? Then are you saying that since that time they have expanded the definition of their use, so to speak, to go beyond what would be classified as a medical condition?

Dr. Edwards. That is exactly correct, yes.

Why don't you stop such advertising? Senator Nelson wanted to know. Was the ad still running?

Dr. Edwards. Dr. Simmons informs me that it is no longer running. We have met with Roche as well as with a number of other manufacturers to correct this type of advertising.

(Indeed, the FDA did take steps to reduce such advertising in a letter sent by Commissioner Edwards. See Figure 9.6.)

Another witness critical of advertising was Dr. Robert Seidenberg, a practicing psychiatrist and professor at New York Upstate Medical Center. Seidenberg (1971) had recently published a harshly critical review of psychotropic drug advertising in *Mental Hygiene* (see Chapter 6), and his testimony was an elaboration of that paper. Much of the blame was laid on the prescribing physician.

In the area of mind drug indoctrination, physicians have been seduced and overwhelmed. As consumers of the first instance, we have been ingenuous, typhoid Marys of drug pandemia. Prone to drug dependence ourselves, we have turned on our client, white, middle-class America—

Regulatory Letter

October 22, 1971

TO ALL SPONSORS OF NEW DRUG APPLICATIONS
FOR PSYCHOTROPIC PRESCRIPTION DRUGS

Gentlemen:

Of growing concern to the Food and Drug Administration is the excessive use of psychotropic prescription drugs for conditions of use that have not been approved and for which there is no substantial proof of efficacy. These drugs are approved for the treatment of clinically significant anxiety, depression, and/or other mental conditions, but, of late, advertisements have also promoted their use in the treatment of symptoms arising from the stresses of everyday living, which cannot properly be defined as pathological.

This communication is to request each sponsor of a psychotropic prescription drug to review all advertising and promotional material for his drug, to determine its compliance with the conditions of use for which the drug is approved. Sponsors are further requested to cancel promptly all advertising and promotion of such drugs which recommend or suggest their use for everyday or minor life stresses, or which are otherwise not in compliance with the conditions of use approved for the drug.

The above information has been supplied to all holders of new drug applications for psychotropic prescription drugs.

Sincerely,

Charles C. Edwards, M.D.
Commissioner of Food and Drugs

FIGURE 9.6

and the kids came tripping after. Physicians are not responsible for all the worldly ills that are the purported reasons for the great drug quest. Nor have we created the life situations that cause patients to plead for relief. Yet we do control out prescription pads and should control our professional organizations and the advertising policies of their journals.

The Kennedy Hearings—Part 1

In 1974, Senator Edward Kennedy's Subcommittee on Health took up the battle in its Examination of the Pharmaceutical Industry, 1973–1974. Among the witnesses was Robert Clark, at that time president of Hoffmann-LaRoche.

Kennedy wanted to know the status of Librium and Valium vis-à-vis the proposal to include them in the list of "controlled substances." (See Drug Abuse Control Amendment Hearings above.) Did Mr. Clark know where that stood?

> Mr. Clark. Yes. After some rather prolonged hearings, what was then the Bureau of Narcotics and Dangerous Drugs, now the DEA, held that they should be placed under control.
>
> We appealed to the Third Circuit, and we won the appeal, but on a procedural point.
>
> It came back to the DEA, Drug Enforcement Administration, and we agreed with them that in view of the long history and the findings in the Third Circuit, if they proposed to list the drugs in Schedule 4, we would not exercise our right of appeal from that finding.
>
> The matter was then referred to the Food and Drug Administration under the law, and at the moment it is still with the Food and Drug Administration.
>
> Senator Kennedy. How long has it been there, do you know?
>
> Mr. Clark. I am not sure exactly, Senator, but several months.
>
> Senator Kennedy. What is your position now with regard to control?
>
> Mr. Clark. What is our position? Well, our position, as I stated, is if DEA proposed to list them in Schedule 4, we will not exercise the right of appeal. My personal feeling is another matter. But that is the practical position we take.
>
> Senator Kennedy. What is your personal feeling?
>
> Mr. Clark. It was a long, vigorously contested proceeding, Senator, and naturally we did not agree with the outcome, but we are prepared to abide by it.

Elsewhere in the hearings, data were presented describing industry practices of providing samples of their products to physicians. Among the data was a listing of samples of certain minor tranquilizers distributed in 1973. These included 122,502 solicited samples of Tranxene (Abbott) mostly in bottles of 30 and something in excess of 175,000 samples of Valium in bottles of 100.

The Nelson Hearings—Part 30

By April 1976, the Nelson Hearings had filled 29 volumes. Volume 30 consisted of testimony, according to Senator Nelson, "concerned with the problem of how the medical profession gets information about drugs and the relationship to prescribing practices, competition and the health and welfare of the public." The major issue was the degree to which medical education, especially postgraduate education was influenced by pharmaceutical manufacturers.

Strong concern was expressed by Dr. Richard Crout, then director of the Bureau of Drugs at the FDA, in his prepared statement.

> There is considerable evidence that the pharmaceutical industry plays a very important, perhaps a dominant, role in the post-graduate education of physicians, dentists, and other health professionals. This role of the pharmaceutical industry in supporting post-graduate medical education has increased rapidly in recent years and, in my opinion, is a problem deserving of national attention.

One of Dr. Crout's concerns was the degree to which the medical journals received by physicians were paid for outright or subsidized by drug advertising. He buttressed his position with the information contained in Table 9.1.

Dr. Crout also had other concerns. One was a symposium sponsored by Wyeth Laboratories that was devoted entirely to its product Serax (oxazepam), a benzodiazepine tranquilizer similar to Librium and Valium. The proceedings of this conference were published as a supplement to the May 1975 issue of *Diseases of the Nervous System*.

> The special issue did not reveal the symposium's sponsorship, but contains articles which suggest special advantages that the Wyeth product may have over the other benzodiazepine tranquilizers.
>
> I want to emphasize again that medical investigators must be free to write whatever they wish about drugs and to speculate about advantages one drug may have over another. In this case, however, the investigators were selected by the manufacturer to participate in an industry-sponsored meeting, the proceedings of the meeting were published without reference to such sponsorship, and the papers all turn out to be favorable to Serax.
>
> Even if the investigators, who are well-known physicians in their field and investigators of known integrity, are accurate in everything they say, the process through which this supplement to a medical publication was produced is cause for concern.

The Kennedy Hearings on Benzodiazepines

On September 9, 1979, Senator Edward Kennedy opened his meeting of the Subcommittee on Health and Scientific Research with the stated purpose "to try to understand the reasons for overuse and misuse of these

TABLE 9.1. Distribution of U.S. Medical Journals with Total Circulation of over 70,000 According to March 24, 1976, Issue of Standard Rate and Data Service

Journal	Free Distribution	Paid Distribution
American Family Physician	108,714	2,307
American Medical News	258,811	
Consultant	142,120	
Current Prescribing	118,168	
Drug Therapy	113,793	
Emergency Medicine	109,974	
Hospital Medicine	178,687	
Hospital Practice	187,134	
Hospital Tribune	100,000	
Infectious Disease	139,840	
Journal of the American Medical Association	27,579	211,856
Journal of Legal Medicine	125,626	
MD Medical Newsmagazine	181,481	
Medical Aspects of Human Sexuality	161,522	
Medical Challenge	77,749	
Medical Economics	169,624	
Medical Opinion	152,191	
Medical Tribune	150,000	
Medical World News	164,652	
Modern Medicine	170,311	
New England Journal of Medicine	923	158,190
Patient Care	101,145	
Physician and Sportsmedicine	90,533	
Physician's Management	179,386	
Postgraduate Medicine	108,068	
Practical Psychology	104,092	
Private Practice	171,659	
Resident and Staff Physician	95,948	319

drugs; to try and alert the American people to the consequences of misuse and abuse; to try to see what can be done to assure appropriate use." The legislation to which the hearing related loosely was the (latest) Drug Regulation Reform Act.

The hearings, conducted by Kennedy along with Senators Schweiker (later secretary of health and human services) and Metzenbaum, began with a panel of witnesses, each with a drug-connected horror story.

- William Thomas, a Long Beach, California, physician who admitted developing a Valium use pattern of more than 50 tablets a day
- William Ryan, a Catholic priest, who described his alcohol and Valium habit as resulting in a condition in which "emptying a waste basket was a week-long project"
- A New Jersey homemaker, Joan Hinton, who obtained Valium prescriptions from four different psychiatrists whom she was seeing simultaneously
- Another homemaker, from Delaware, who repeated that her psychiatrist advised her that she needed Valium in the same way a diabetic needs insulin
- A female bank officer from California who decided she was addicted to Valium after watching a "60 Minutes" program
- A meter reader from Atlanta who described in a rather fuzzy fashion his long years of using drugs and alcohol
- Another physician, from North Carolina, who supplied the most quotable, and quoted, line of the hearings: "While all the other doctors in Boston were reading their morning mail, I would be eating mine."

Testimony was heard from Robert Clark, president of Hoffmann-LaRoche, who was accompanied by Roche Medical Director Bruce Medd, Dr. Leo Hollister of Stanford, Dr. David Smith of the Haight-Ashbury Clinic, and physician-writer Michael Halberstam.

Clark opened his testimony with the observation that "the first panel [of witnesses at the hearing] unquestionably involved the most classic disobeyance of the package insert that I have ever heard in my life." He and Kennedy then engaged in a dialogue dealing with package inserts and the addictive properties of Valium.

Dr. Halberstam saw the effects of the hearings in a dangerous light. "I think the thrust of these hearings so far is to add an additional burden of guilt and anxiety to these people who are genuinely, albeit usually temporarily, overwhelmed."

Considerable attention was also devoted to the so-called Cornell Stress Program. This three-year program, which cost Roche nearly $5 million, resulted from a grant to Health Learning Systems, which in turn dealt with Cornell Provost for Medical Affairs Theodore Cooper. The major issue that formed the theme of these discussions was whether Roche (through Health Learning Systems) was attempting to "teach" physicians about stress while suggesting that stress was an indication for Valium.

Senator Metzenbaum was especially concerned about the Cornell Program.

Senator Metzenbaum. Mr. Chairman, before we return to Mr. Clark, I would like to get a comment on the testimony that was given before. Dr. Medd said that when Cornell's study was made, they mentioned many of the various tranquilizers, and my understanding is that Cornell Medical School sent out 80,000 cassettes of an interview of Ed Newman with Dr. Theodore Cooper, who headed up this program.

You could not have read anything that was more of a push for Valium than the statements that are made in that particular transcript of the cassette. I find nowhere that any other medicines are mentioned.

Mr. Newman says, "Today, we will be discussing that program, the benefits of that program to improve patient care." Dr. Cooper then responds to Mr. Newman some pages later, "On the one hand, we have the scientific and clinical research and the literature, which, over the many years, have established the safety and reliability of Valium and some of the other benzodiazepines."

Mr. Newman says, "Do the risks outweigh the benefits?" Cooper: "Definitely not, in my opinion. The benefits usually greatly exceed the risks, even though millions of benzodiazepine tablets and capsules, such as Valilum, have been prescribed to millions of patients over the years." At various other points, Valium is mentioned.

Now, what concerns me, Mr. Clark, is that you head up a very responsible and respected company; you have a good reputation in the industry. Is there not some sense of impropriety in spending over $4 million to fund a program at Cornell which, in essence, winds up being nothing more than a kind of medical approval, which is merchandised and marketed by your company?

Is there not something wrong with that kind of procedure? You give $4 million and you get all this extra push for your product.

Mr. Clark. Let me reiterate again that we have absolutely no control over what Dr. Cooper says.

Senator Metzenbaum. Mr. Clark, do you not think that when you give somebody $4 million to head up a program and they wind up saying all the right things about your product—you do not have to say, "Now, Dr. Cooper, you have to remember to say it this way." It is obvious. He said it that way, for $4 million.

Mr. Clark. Senator Metzenbaum, you are a terrible cynic, I am afraid. I know Dr. Cooper and I think he is a very reliable, honest man. He happens to mention Valium, because that is what everybody talks about when they are talking about minor tranquilizers.

Senator Metzenbaum. And Valium happens to be the one funding the program, am I right?

Senator Kennedy's summary of the reports from this panel included the observations that (1) Valium is addictive, but patients and physicians may not be aware of that; (2) The withdrawal aspects are "extremely harsh"; and (3) It is possible to free oneself from the Valium addiction.

The hearings continued with statements from a panel of scientists and physicians who generally agreed that addiction to Valium and other tranquilizers was a real phenomenon, that the drugs were overprescribed, and that a partial cause of the overprescribing was failure of physicians to recognize the dangers of the drugs.

Then Director of the Bureau of Drugs (FDA) Richard Crout was the next to testify. His testimony addressed several issues. Among them were

1. New warning labeling for the benzodiazepines using the words "psychological and physical dependence" (according to Crout, a more precise term for addiction).
2. A Roche-sponsored medical education program on the consequences of stress.
3. Patient package inserts.

Included among the materials supplied along with Dr. Crout's prepared statement was an interesting internal memo from Thomas Hayes, chief of the FDA Psychopharmacology Unit, discussing the proposed changes in labeling:

> There is another area of concern with diazepam labeling unrelated to the recent correspondence regarding dependents, i.e., the wording in the INDICATIONS section which states that "diazepam is useful in the symptomatic relief of tension and anxiety states resulting from stressful circumstances or whenever symptomatic complaints are concomitants of emotional factors." In view of the recent attention generated by the Roche Symposium on Stress, I am concerned that the inclusion of this wording in the INDICATION section of one (but not all) of the benzodiazepines might prove to be a commercial advantage for which FDA might be considered responsible. Other products, e.g., Wyeth's Ativan (lorazepam), utilize terminology such as transient situational disturbances which I find preferable.

Ultimately, as testimony showed, the Valium package insert was changed to read as follows: "Valium is indicated for the symptomatic relief of anxiety and tension associated with anxiety disorders, transient situational disturbances and functional or organic disorders."

Crout commented on criticism of the level of use of the benzodiazepines:

> Whether benzodiazepines are, in fact, overprescribed relative to medical need, however, is a question that cannot be answered with scientific certainty. The fundamental reason for this difficulty is that because of differing value judgments on how best to treat patients with anxiety or

tension, there is no consensus on how to establish the optimal medical need for these drugs. The problem is further complicated by imprecision in the diagnosis of psychoneurotic disorders and lack of good epidemiological data on the extent and duration of benzodiazepine use in various subgroups of the general population.

He noted also that "the benzodiazepines are very useful and important drugs in modern medicine. They have undoubtedly helped millions of people with anxiety and tension. Given their wide usage, they have also had a remarkable safety record."

Among the documents presented by Crout was the 1971 letter from FDA Commissioner Edwards asking all tranquilizer manufacturers to tone down their promotions (see Figure 9.6).

Kennedy's committee also solicited and received a detailed communication from the National Consumers League. Their recommendations went much further than actions taken by FDA, and are listed below. There is little evidence of any action on any of these recommendations.

(1) Move to correct excessive use of Valium and Librium through an extensive consumer and doctor educational program. Patient package inserts must be included for Valium, Librium and all drugs. The package inserts must be written by an objective panel, not the industry, and they must state clearly the dangers associated with the drugs.

(2) Doctors must stop prescribing Valium and Librium on a "Use as Needed" basis.

(3) Senior citizens must be told that the dosages of Valium and Librium which they are receiving are established for young men, and therefore may not be appropriate for elderly people. Incalculable damage including possible brain damage has been recorded because of the failure to adjust dosages for the age of the population receiving them.

(4) The two drugs should be removed from their special Schedule IV and placed on a more restrictive schedule. This will help solve the problem of doctors thinking Valium and Librium are less dangerous than other addictive drugs.

(5) FDA should initiate a series of nationwide hearings at which consumers can testify on the deleterious effects of Valium and Librium. All expenses, including travel, expert witness fees, childcare, and legal counsel must be paid for by FDA at these hearings.

(6) Now that the seventeen year patent has or is expiring on Valium and Librium, FDA should launch a national campaign urging that they be known by their generic names diazepam and cholordiazepoxide hydrochloride. Only in that way can Hoffmann-LaRoche's stranglehold on the market be lessened.

(7) If Valium and Librium are to be included in any formulary which
FDA recommends for coverage under national health insurance,
appropriate and adequate warnings about the potential dangers of
the drug must be included.

The hearing adjourned after approximately four hours, but generated 525
pages of testimony, prepared statements, and supporting material.

Senator Nelson—Reprise

Within 10 days of the conclusion of the Kennedy Hearings, Senator
Nelson's Select Committee on Small Business published an "analysis and
review of the psychotropic drug hearings" that had been conducted at
various times by his Subcommittee on Monopoly and Anticompetitive
Activities. The report had been prepared by the Congressional Research
Service.*

According to the report, the policy issues raised during the course of
the various hearings included

the lack of adequate physician education in pharmacology; the responsibility of the consumer, the prescribing physician, and the medical
community for the problem of psychotropic drug overuse; governmental
regulation of drug use; and the need for more research and researchers to
study psychotropic drugs, their risks and benefits.

The Wolff Hearings—1979

The final congressional hearings conducted during this period were
those of the Select Committee on Narcotics Abuse and Control, chaired by
Lester L. Wolff (New York). Testimony and materials submitted were
summarized in a 1979 report from the committee.

The report began with a listing of "Findings Relating to Psychotropics
and A.M.A." The list of 25 items serves as a convenient summary of the
work of prior hearings.

1. Retail prescriptions for antianxiety agents have more than
doubled since 1964, to cover 100 million annually.
2. The Food and Drug Administration (FDA) reviewed 26,843

---

*The report provides a good review of the substance of the respective hearings in
somewhat more detail than is provided in this chapter and offers a valuable topical index and
list of witnesses.

advertising and promotional labeling items in 1977. Of this number only 97 were the subject of FDA regulatory actions.

3. The Pharmaceutical Manufacturers Association (PMA) sees few faults with the drug advertising in professional journals and defends the material as representing "average patients". The PMA has thus rarely initiated an investigation into the way a product is advertised.

4. The PMA admitted that psychotropic drugs provide only symptomatic relief and not cure.

5. The problem of licit drug abuse or overdose is often hidden.

6. The number of people affected by the problem of misuse or abuse of licit drugs is larger than those who abuse illegal drugs.

7. The physician is the primary channel of distribution for licit prescription drugs.

8. The American Medical Association (AMA) has no formal mechanism for dealing with physicians who overprescribe.

9. No effective action has been taken by the AMA to review the credentials of physicians indicted for questionable professional practices.

10. The AMA does not consider physicians having financial interests in pharmacies as having a conflict of interest.

11. The national AMA does not control membership criteria at the local level.

12. The AMA does not view overprescribing or misprescribing a serious enough national problem to treat it as a crisis in the medical profession.

13. Legitimate medical need for psychotropic drugs is difficult to assess. Domestic shipments of central nervous system drugs (of which psychotropic drugs are a part) rose from $518 million to $986 million in the 10-year period ending 1975. This constitutes an alarming increase unless it can be demonstrated that the increased volume of sales is in response to a corresponding increase in legitimate medical need.

14. Illicit consumption of amphetamines has been greatly reduced as a direct result of their being placed on schedule II of the Controlled Substances Act.

15. The pharmaceutical industry appears to increase the demand for as much of their drug products as possible, regardless of the real need for such products.

16. Advertising in medical journals is one of the prime means employed by the pharmaceutical industry to sell its products. In

1978, the pharmaceutical industry spent approximately $566 million for product promotion. Included in this figure was $266 million for detail people and $131 million for direct mailing, sampling, and journal advertising.

17. The primary purpose of the pharmaceutical industry's promotional expenditures is to persuade physicians to prescribe one product over competing products.

18. The promotional activities of the pharmaceutical companies are the major influence upon physicians in determining their prescribing practices.

19. A study in California found that 3 percent of the patients are shopping and abusing the legal drug prescription model for 50 percent of the time it is being abused. The remaining abuse is initiated by some physicians who indiscriminately prescribe and are thus in the business of selling prescriptions for dangerous drugs.

20. Prior to offering other products, Roche asks its detail people, upon visiting physicians, to first present Valium.

21. Hoffmann-LaRoche (Roche) applies considerable pressure upon their detail people to increase sales. Quotas (called "goals") are established for sales of Valium and detail people are expected to meet or exceed these standards.

22. In 1977 Roche had sales revenue of $370 million. Valium, a minor tranquilizer and the single most popular drug in the United States, accounted for $250 million of this total.

23. In 1977 Roche expended $40 million on advertising; $9 million upon Valium.

24. Although the majority of detail people at Roche have graduated from high school and/or college and many have a degree in one of the sciences, Roche has no minimal education requirement for its detail people.

25. Computer technology has advanced to the stage where terminals in pharmacies linked to a central computer could provide a means of drug utilization review thus minimizing abuse from this source. Problems still exist as to issues of financing, confidentiality, concept, and coordination, but the time is approaching when some model of drug utilization review must be implemented.

Because the Wolff Hearings were the last of the period and presumably benefited from information previously generated, the conclusions and recommendations are reproduced here.

CONCLUSIONS

1. The pharmaceutical industry appears to try to sell as much of their drug products as possible regardless of the "real" need for such products. In so doing, they use pressure sales tactics that have been highly successful. Profit statements, net sales, and number of kilos and capsules of drugs produced are closely guarded industry secrets.

2. The sales tactics employed by the pharmaceutical industry help create a questionable market and a demand for psychotropic drugs. This is often done by finding "wider" indications for drugs that were earlier marketed for "narrow" uses. As a result of these kinds of sales tactics, the demand, and indeed, the misuse of psychotropic drugs have reached what could legitimately be called epidemic proportions.

3. The widespread prescribing of psychotropic medication and psychotherapeutic agents by all areas of medical specialties poses a threat to the health of the American public.

4. The pharmaceutical industry seems unwilling to set limits on the amount of psychoactive drugs that they manufacture. They appear unwilling to monitor their own distribution system. They, in effect, place the blame for any overprescribing and over-utilization of psychotropics that might exist upon the American people.

5. The pharmaceutical industry's entire promotional effort as to psychotropic drugs is directed toward the physician, the pharmacy, and the hospital formulary. Toward these ends pharmaceutical detailmen are extensively trained in how to contact and personally indoctrinate physicians as to the merits of their products. One company, Roche, from testimony taken, asks its detail people to promote Valium first, the leading selling prescription drug in the United States, upon any visit to a physician or pharmacy. This approach is yet another indication of the primary objective of the industry—to sell its products and increase profits, while inadequately fulfilling their responsibility to meet the public trust.

6. Information regarding the psychopharmacologic aspects of psychotropic drugs and their place in medical practice is heavily influenced by the pharmaceutical inudstry. In effect, detailment become educators of physicians, pharmacists, and other health professionals who accept responsibility for dispensing drugs to the American public. Testimony on postgraduate creidt hours to physicians did not convince the committee that medical profes-

sionals were gaining sufficiently in their education from this source. It was concluded that the industry heavily influenced both the kind of information and the amount of information disseminated in pharmacologic education courses to physicians and in fact often provided their logo in various training devices given to physicians.

7. Pharmacologic and psychopharmacologic information recieved by the physician through the pharmaceutical industry far outweighs that which he or she may obtain through formal medical education. The Physicians' Desk Reference and the drug industry apparently serve as the major influence in guiding the physician's prescribing practices.

8. The physician has the primary responsibility to ensure the rational use of psychoactive medications by his patients. It is concluded from testimony that many physicians do not take adequate time to properly enumerate efficacy and safety issues when they dispense psychoactive medications.

9. Some physicians have not undertaken sufficient responsibility in the proper prescribing and dispensing of psychoactive substances. Testimony given to this committee indicates that there are those physicians who are guided in their prescribing practices by the patient, that is, some physicians dispense psychoactive medication in order to keep the patient "happy" and enable him to end an office visit in a "reasonable" length of time.

10. Testimony by the Pharmaceutical Manufacturers Association indicates that the industry has not accepted their full responsibility for improper, illicit, or overutilization of psychotropic substances. In this regard, the industry seems to lay the blame for such abuses at the feet of the American public.

RECOMMENDATIONS AS TO PSYCHOTROPICS AND THE AMA

1. The Congress must continue to encourage the AMA to establish a committee within the organization to provide effective oversight of the prescribing practices of physicians. Failing that, the medical profession may be faced with imposed regulatory requirements.

2. The Congress should enact legislation to impose a nominal tax on the manufacture of psychoactive substances with the revenue so raised used to support an extensive education and prevention program.

3. Congress should encourage the pharmaceutical industry to develop and implement programs of drug education for physicians

and consumers. There should be a particular emphasis placed on special population groups, women, elderly, youth and minorities.

4. Congress should encourage the pharmaceutical industry to develop education and training standards for detailment. This training should include a definite number of hours in clinical pharmacology, drug chemistry, human anatomy, and ethical sales procedures.

5. The FDA has been reluctant to intrude upon the doctor-patient relationship. In the case of methadone, however, it was determined that the absence of tight control of the distribution of the drug would constitute a threat to the public health. Accordingly, FDA requires a special license be issued to any individual or organization dispensing methadone. It is the recommendation of the Select Committee that similar licensing requirements be required for the outpatient distributor of amphetamines and short-acting barbiturates (barbiturate hypnotics).

6. An advisory council of eminent psychopharmacologists, physicians, and pharmacists should be established by the FDA. The council should set an upper limit on the dosage units of various psychotropic drugs that may be dispensed to an outpatient at any one time. These limits shall be then incorporated into the law.

7. Testimony revealed a small minority of patients who doctor and/ or pharmacy shop, that is they may receive multiple prescriptions from several physicians and have them filled at several different pharmacies. One answer to this type of diversion is drug utilization review. This could be accomplished through terminals in all pharmacies linked to a central computer file. We recommend that the feasibility of such a system be explored and perhaps pilot tested. The committee recommends that NIDA make funds available for the appropriate research.

8. Drug Investigation Units (DIU's) have been relatively successful in their efforts against "script" doctors in California. It is therefore recommended that the possibility of expanding the role of DIU's to include comprehensive monitoring of prescriptions be examined by DEA and other agencies involved.

9. The Drug Regulation Reform Act which failed passage at the end of the 95th Congress included language that would have placed a limitation on the distribution of controlled drugs. It is recommended that provisions be added to this legislation which will require dosage limitations on the prescriptions of certain scheduled drugs.

10. The committee recommends that a "model Health Professions Practice Act and State Regulatory Policy" be adopted and

implemented by each State. The act provides maximum freedom to health professionals while at the same time providing a system of checks, safeguards, and sanctions, to minimize abuse.

11. The committee recommends that legislation be passed to require notification to DEA of all prescriptions involving controlled substances above a minimal dosage amount so as to regulate the indiscriminate distribution of chemicals of abuse.

12. Drug companies which manufacture dangerous drugs not yet under State and Federal control should carefully monitor their sales and those of their customers to assure that:

    (a) Inordinate amounts are not passed through channels of trade so as to foster possible street use.

    (b) They know on a daily basis where their dangerous products are being sold and dispensed by physicians.

    (c) They are in a position to alert law enforcement officials at the first signs of diversion, overprescribing, or overdispensing.

    (d) They assume more responsibility to the public at large since they are profiting from the sales of substances inherently dangerous to humans.

THE FOOD AND DRUG ADMINISTRATION

The FDA is, of course, the single federal agency with the greatest responsibility for prescription drugs. It monitors the research process and the marketing of such medications, having responsibility for manufacture and promotion as well. Within this function, the FDA has dealt with the minor tranquilizers since they first appeared.

Though the FDA's regulator activities are direct, its influence is often subtle, especially insofar as it must approve the final official labeling of all prescription drugs. This labeling specifies, in detail, the approved use of drugs and, by regulation, serves as the official reference point against which to judge the content of promotional messages.

The 1962 Drug Amendments serve as the point at which the FDA began to "flex its muscles" (indeed, the amendments gave the FDA the muscles) regarding promotion. This point is well illustrated by an examination of product descriptions from the *Physicians' Desk Reference* (*PDR*). The *PDR* product descriptions, while not "official," must pass FDA supervision and thus serve as a convenient source of comparison. We have reproduced *PDR* descriptions of meprobamate (as Miltown) for selected years to illustrate labeling changes undertaken at FDA request (Figures 9.7, 9.8, 9.9).

MILTOWN^R

COMPOSITION: Meprobamate Wallace (2-methyl-2-n-propyl-1, 3-propanediol dicarbamate).

ACTION AND USES: An entirely new tranquilizer with muscle relaxant action, for control of anxiety and tension, and muscular spasm. Blocks interneuronal hyperactivity; selectively synchronizes E.E.G. potentials from the thalamus. For restored tranquility in anxiety and tension states, for sleeplessness due to worry, and for muscle spasm, particularly in fibrositic conditions. Also indicated in idiopathic minor epilepsies and for relaxation of muscle tension in some cases of cerebral palsy. Ineffective in Parkinson's disease, grand mal, and rheumatoid arthritis. Miltown acts on the central nervous system only; does not affect autonomic functions. Essentially nontoxic. Side effects minimal.

ADMINISTRATION AND DOSAGE: Fully effective on oral administration; 1 or 2 tablets, three times a day; for sleep, 2 tablets, before retiring.

HOW SUPPLIED: 400 mg. scored tablets bottles of 50.

FIGURE 9.7. Description of Miltown, from the 1957 *Physicians' Desk Reference.*

MILTOWN[R]

[Shown in Product Identification Section]

COMPOSITION: Meprobamate Wallace (2-methyl-2-n-propyl-1, 3-propanediol dicarbamate).

ACTION AND USES: Tranquilizer with muscle relaxant action, for control of anxiety, tension and skeletal muscle spasm. Blocks interneuronal hyperactivity; selectively synchronizes E.E.G. potentials from the thalamus. For restored tranquility in anxiety and tension states, pre- and post-operative care, for sleeplessness due to worry, and for muscle spasm, particularly in fibrositic conditions. Also indicated in idiopathic minor epilepsies and for relaxation of muscle tension in some cases of cerebral palsy. Ineffective in Parkinson's disease, grand mal, and rheumatoid arthritis. MILTOWN acts on the central nervous system only; does not affect autonomic functions. Essentially nontoxic. Side effects minimal.

ADMINISTRATION AND DOSAGE: Fully effective on oral administration; one or two 400 mg. tablets, three times a day; for sleep, 2 tablets, before retiring.

PRECAUTIONS: Careful supervision of dose and amounts of meprobamate prescribed for patients is advised; especially with those patients with a known propensity for taking excessive quantities of drugs. Excessive and prolonged use in susceptible persons has been reported to result in dependence on the drug. Where excessive dosage has continued for weeks or months, dosage should be reduced gradually rather than abruptly stopped, since sudden withdrawal may precipitate withdrawal reactions. These have in some cases taken the form of epileptiform seizures.

HOW SUPPLIED: 400 mg. scored tablets and 200 mg. sugar-coated tablets, bottles of 50.

LITERATURE AVAILABLE: Yes.

FIGURE 9.8. Description of Miltown, from the 1961 *Physicians'
Desk Reference.*

MILTOWN/MILTOWN 600
(meprobamate/meprobamate 600 mg.)

Description: Meprobamate is a white powder with a characteristic odor and a
bitter taste. It is slightly soluble in water, freely soluble in acetone and alcohol,
and sparingly soluble in ether.

Actions: Meprobamate is a carbamate derivative which has been shown in
animal studies to have effects at multiple sites in the central nervous system,
including the thalamus and limbic system.

Indication: Meprobamate is indicated for the relief of anxiety and tension; as an
adjunct in the treatment of various disease states in which anxiety and tension
are manifested; and to promote sleep in anxious tense patients. The effectiveness
of 'Miltown' in long-term use, that is, more than 4 months, has not been assessed
by systematic clinical studies. The physician should periodically reassess the
usefulness of the drug for the individual patient.

Contraindications: Acute intermittent porphyria as well as allergic or idiosyncratic reactions to meprobamate or related compounds such as carisoprodol,
mebutamate, tybamate, or carbromal.

Warnings:
Drug Dependence
Physical dependence, psychological dependence, and abuse have occurred. When
chronic intoxication from prolonged use occurs, it usually involves ingestion of
greater than recommended doses and is manifested by ataxia, slurred speech, and
vertigo. Therefore, careful supervision of dose and amounts prescribed is advised,
as well as avoidance of prolonged administration, especially for alcoholics and
other patients with a known propensity for taking excessive quantities of drugs.
Sudden withdrawal of the drug after prolonged and excessive use may precipitate
recurrence of preexisting symptoms, such as anxiety, anorexia, or insomnia, or
withdrawal reactions, such as vomiting, ataxia, tremors, muscle twitching, con-
fusional states, hallucinosis, and, rarely, convulsive seizures. Such seizures are
more likely to occur in persons with central nervous system damage or pre-
existent or latent convulsive disorders. Onset of withdrawal symptoms occurs
usually within 12 to 48 hours after discontinuation of meprobamate; symptoms
usually cease within the next 12 to 48 hours. When excessive dosage has
continued for weeks or months, dosage should be reduced gradually over a
period of one or two weeks rather than abruptly stopped. Alternatively, a short-
acting barbiturate may be substituted, then gradually withdrawn.

Potentially Hazardous Tasks
Patients should be warned that this drug may impair the mental and/or physical

FIGURE 9.9. Description of Miltown, from the 1980 *Physicians'*
Desk Reference.

abilities required for the performance of potentially hazardous tasks such as driving a motor vehicle or operating machinery.

Addictive Effects
Since the effects of meprobamate and alcohol or meprobamate and other CNS depressants or psychotropic drugs may be addictive, appropriate caution should be exercised with patients who take more than one of these agents simultaneously.

Usage in Pregnancy and Lactation
An increased risk of congenital malformations associated with the use of minor tranquilizers (meprobamate, chlordiazepoxide, and diazepam) during the first trimester of pregnancy has been suggested in several studies. Because use of these drugs is rarely a matter of urgency, their use during this period should always be avoided. The possibility that a woman of childbearing potential may be pregnant at the time of institution of therapy should be considered. Patients should be advised that if they become pregnant during therapy or intend to become pregnant they should communicate with their physicians about the desirability of discontinuing the drug. Meprobamate passes the placental barrier. It is present both in umbilical cord blood at or near maternal plasma levels and in breast milk of lactating mothers at concentrations two to four times that of maternal plasma. When use of meprobamate is contemplated in breast-feeding patients, the milk as compared to maternal plasma levels should be considered.

Usage in Children—Meprobamate should not be administered to children under age six, since there is a lack of documented evidence for safety and effectiveness in this age group.
'Miltown' 600 (meprobamate 600 mg.)—This dosage form is not intended for use in children.
Precautions: The lowest effective dose should be administered, particularly to elderly and/or debilitated patients, in order to preclude oversedation. The possibility of suicide attempts should be considered and the least amount of drug feasible should be dispensed at any one time. Meprobamate is metabolized in the liver and excreted by the kidney; to avoid its excess accumulation, caution should be exercised in administration to patients with compromised liver or kidney function. Meprobamate occasionally may precipitate seizures in epileptic patients.
Adverse Reactions:
Central Nervous System
Drowsiness, ataxia, dizziness, slurred speech, headache, vertigo, weakness, paresthesias, impairment of visual accommodation, euphoria, overstimulation, paradoxical excitement, fast EEG activity.
Gastrointestinal
Nausea, vomiting, diarrhea.
Cardiovascular

(continued)

Palpitations, tachycardia, various forms of arrhythmia, transient ECG changes, syncope; also, hypotensive crises (including one fatal case).

Allergic or Idiosyncratic

Allergic or idiosyncratic reactions are usually seen within the period of the first to fourth dose in patients having no previous contact with the drug. Milder reactions are characterized by an itchy, urticarial, or erythematous maculopapular rash which may be generalized or confined to the groin. Other reactions have included leukopenia, acute nonthrombocytopenic purpura, petachiae, ecchymoses, eosinophilia, peripheral edema, adenopathy, fever, fixed drug eruption with cross reaction to carisoprodo, and cross sensitivity between meprobamate/ mebutamate and meprobamate/carbromal. More severe hypersensitivity reactions, rarely reported, include hyperpyrexia, chills, angioneurotic edema, bronchospasm, oliguria, and anuria. Also anaphylaxis, erythema multiforme, exfoliative dermatitis, stomatitis, proctitis, Stevens-Johnson syndrome, and bullous dermatitis, including one fatal case of the latter following administration of meprobamate in combination with prednisolone. In case of allergic or idiosyncratic reactions to meprobamate, discontinue the drug and initiate appropriate symptomatic therapy, which may include epinephrine, antihistamines, and in severe cases, corticosteroids. In evaluating possible allergic reactions, also consider allergy to excipients (information on excipients is available to physicians on request).

(See also Allergic or Idiosyncratic.) Agranulocytosis and aplastic anemia have been reported, although no causal relationship has been established. These cases rarely were fatal. Rare cases of thrombocytopenic purpura have been reported.

Other

Exacerbation of prophyric symptoms.

Dosage and Administration

Adults: 'Miltown' (meprobamate)—the usual dosage is 1200 to 1600 mg daily administered in three or four divided doses.

'Miltown' 600 (meprobamate 600 mg)—the recommended dosage is one tablet twice a day. Doses of meprobamate about 2400 mg daily are not recommended.

Children: 'Miltown' (meprobamate)—the usual dosage for children ages six to twelve is 100 to 200 mg two or three times daily. Meprobamate is not recommended for children under six.

'Miltown' 600 (meprobamate 600 mg)—is not intended for use in children.

Overdosage: Suicide attempts with meprobamate have resulted in drowsiness, lethargy, stupor, ataxia, coma, shock, vasomotor and respiratory collapse. Some suicidal attempts have been fatal. The following data on meprobamate tablets have been reported in the literature and from other sources. These data are not expected to correlate with each case (considering factors such as individual susceptibility and length of time from ingestion to treatment), but represent the usual ranges reported.

Acute simple overdose (meprobamate alone): Death has been reported with ingestion of as little as 12 gm meprobamate and survival with as much as 40 gm.

FIGURE 9.9. (continued)

Blood Levels

0.5–2.0 mg% represents the usual blood level range of meprobamate after therapeutic doses. The level may occasionally be as high as 3.0 mg%.

3–10 mg% usually corresponds to findings of mild to moderate symptoms of overdosage, such as stupor or light coma.

10–20 mg% usually corresponds to deeper coma, requiring more intensive treatment. Some fatalities occur.

At levels greater than 20 mg%, more fatalities than survivals can be expected. Acute combined overdose (meprobamate with alcohol or other CNS depressants or psychotropic drugs): Since effects can be addictive a history of ingestion or a low dose of meprobamate plus any of these compounds (or of a relatively low blood or tissue level) cannot be used as a prognostic indicator. In cases where excessive doses have been taken, sleep ensues rapidly and blood pressure, pulse, and respiratory rates are reduced to basal levels. Any drug remaining in the stomach should be removed and symptomatic therapy given. Should respiration or blood pressure become compromised, respiratory assistance, central nervous system stimulants, and pressor agents should be administered cautiously as indicated. Meprobamate is metabolized in the liver and excreted by the kidney. Diuresis, osmotic (mannitol) diuresis, peritoneal dialysis, and hemodialysis have been used successfully. Careful monitoring of urinary output is necessary and caution should be taken to avoid overhydration. Relapse and death, after initial recovery have been attributed to incomplete gastric emptying and delaying absorption. Meprobamate can be measured in biological fluids by two methods: colorimetric (Hoffman, A. J. and Ludwig, B. J.: J. Amer. Pharm. Assn. 48:740, 1959) and gas chromatographic (Douglas, J. F. et al: Anal. Chem. 39:956, 1967).

How supplied: 'Miltown' (meprobamate, US.P.) is available as:

−400 mg. white, scored tablets in bottles of
    100 (NDC 0037–1001–01)
    500 (NDC 0037–1001–03)
    1000 (NDC 0037–1001–02)
−200 mg. white sugar-coated tablets in bottles of
    100 (NDC 0037–1101–01)

The 1957 Miltown description is short, indeed. It differs from the 1961 description in deletion of reference to its being "new" and substantively by the addition in the 1961 description of a section on precautions. The 1980 version illustrates dramatically the effect of the 1962 Amendments and subsequent FDA regulations. It is fully six times the length of the 1957 version, and now contains strong warnings on dependence, long-term use, and use in pregnancy. By 1980 Wyeth had chosen not to include a full description in the *PDR* for Equanil, preferring instead to refer the physician to a member of the sales staff.

The 1961 Librium description in the *PDR* was quite extensive, even prior to the forthcoming FDA requirements. The 1980 version had virtually doubled in size and changed considerably in content. Gone was a statement that the product was "virtually specific." Although described as "among the safer pharmacologic compounds," the description contained new warnings about use in pregnancy and the possibility of "paradoxical reactions."

On September 10, 1979, Crout told the Kennedy Committee that the FDA was revising the labeling on benzodiazepines to remove the indications of "stress and stressful situations." On November 21, the FDA wrote the four manufacturers affected (Roche, Librium and Valium; Wyeth, Ativan and Serax; Abbott, Tranxene; Warner Chilcott, Verstran) and asked them to substitute new labeling in the indications section of the approved labeling.

The new labeling, which received FDA approval for the changes in late May 1980, contained a revised indication that stated, "[drug name] is indicated for the management of anxiety disorders or for the short-term relief of the symptoms of anxiety. Anxiety or tension associated with the stress of everyday life usually does not require treatment with an anxiolytic."

The version differed from an earlier agency revision by consolidating the first two sentences of that version and deleting references to anxiety "associated with significant transient situational disturbances" or "with physical illness (e.g. myocardial infarction)." The new revision also substituted "anxiety" for "mild anxiety." Public reports of the labeling chnages were a cause of concern to Roche, which felt that the change was "interpreted by the press as applying to Valium more so than any other minor tranquilizers." FDA Public Affairs Associate Commissioner Wayne Pines replied that Valium "has become almost a generic name for minor tranquilizers so that the press reaction was natural. The market leader not only garners the money, but also the criticism" (FDC Reports 1980a).

"Valium's anxiolytic adjunctive treatment of serious disorders accounts for 65–70% of its use," Roche pointed out in response to publicity generated by the FDA's July 10 press announcement of its recent changes in benzodiazepine labeling. "Approximately 30–35% of the Valium use is for the management of anxiety disorders uncomplicated by other observable medical problems," Roche said. "The remaining 65–70% is used adjunctively for the treatment of anxiety and tension related to serious organic or functional disorders such as cardiovascular or gastrointestinal problems, muscle disorders and certain convulsive diseases."

While expressing support for the label changes, Roche cited a 1975 study, conducted "with the support and cooperation" of the NIMH, to counter the suggestion "that tranquilizers are being used indiscriminately to

Examine Me.

During the past several years, I have heard my name mentioned in movies, on television and radio talk shows, and even at Senate subcommittee sessions. And I have seen it repeatedly in newspapers, magazines, and yes, best-sellers. Lately, whenever I see or hear the phrases "overmedicated society," "overuse," "misuse," and "abuse," my name is one of the reference points. Sometimes even *the* reference point.

These current issues, involving patient compliance or dependency-proneness, should be given careful scrutiny, for they may impede my overall therapeutic usefulness. As you know, a problem almost always involves improper usage. When I am prescribed and taken correctly, I can produce the effective relief for which I am intended.

Amid all this controversy, I ask you to reflect on and re-examine my merits. Think back on the patients in your practice who have been helped through your clinical counseling and prudent prescriptions for me. Consider your patients with heart problems, G.I. problems, and inter-personal problems who, when their anxiety was severe, have been able to benefit from the medication choice you've made. Recall how often you've heard, as a result, "Doctor, I don't know what I would have done without your help."

You and I can feel proud of what we've done together to reduce excessive anxiety and thus help patients to cope more successfully.

If you examine and evaluate me in the light of your own experience, you'll come away with a confirmation of your knowledge that I *am* a safe and effective drug when prescribed judiciously and used wisely.

For a brief summary of product information on Valium (diazepam/ Roche) ℞, please see the following page. Valium is available as 2-mg, 5-mg and 10-mg scored tablets.

FIGURE 9.10

deal with the everyday anxiety of living." The study showed "that this is not the case," the company maintained.

FDA Commissioner Goyan's announcement of the new labeling—which was first indicated in the agency's late May approval of several manufacturers' revised labels—was in keeping with his oft-expressed concern about "overmedication." The FDA press release announcement of the labeling change got wide lay-press treatment at the end of the week of July 11, 1980.

Feelings vs.

*Some people feel that I am misused and overused
and that I'm prescribed too often and for too many kinds
of problems.*

The FACT is that approximately eight million people,
or about 5 percent of the U.S. adult population, will use me
during the current year. By contrast, the national health
examination survey (1971-1975) found that 25 percent of
the U.S. adult population experiences moderate to severe
psychological distress. Additionally, studies of patient attitudes revealed that most patients have realistic views regarding the limitations of tranquilizers and a strong conservatism
about their use, as evidenced by a general tendency to
*de*crease intake over time. Finally, a six-year, large-scale,
carefully conducted national survey showed that the great
majority of physicians appropriately prescribe tranquilizers.

*Some people feel that patients being treated with anxiolytic
drugs are "weak," can't tolerate the anxieties of normal daily
living, and should be able to resolve their problems on their
own without the help of medication.*

The FACT is that while most people can withstand
normal, everyday anxieties, some people experience
excessive and persistent levels of anxiety due to personal or
clinical problems. An extensive national survey concluded
that Americans who do use tranquilizers have substantial

FIGURE 9.11

"I hope MDs adhere closely to these revised indications and become
more discriminating in prescribing tranquilizers to relieve the symptoms of
anxiety," Goyan said. "I hope too that patients will not pressure their MDs
for drugs that are clearly not needed. Tranquilizers can do great good in
helping people get through crisis situations or in helping with problems of
mental illness. Yet millions of Americans are taking them habitually just to
deal with the anxiety of living."

One of the most interesting developments in the advertising/regulatory
arena was the Roche ad campaign, begun in 1981, for Valium. Two ads,

Facts

justification as evidenced by their high levels of anxiety. It was further noted that antianxiety drugs are not usually prescribed for trivial, transient emotional problems.

Some people feel afraid of me because of the stories they've heard about my being harmful and having the potential to produce physical dependence.

The FACT is that there are thousands of references in the medical literature documenting my efficacy and safety. Extensive and painstakingly thorough studies of toxicological data conclude that I am one of the safest types of psychotropic drugs available. Moreover, I do not cause physical dependence if the recommended dosage and therapeutic regimen are followed under careful physician supervision. — DELETED
However, I can produce dependence if patients do not follow their physicians' directions and take me for prolonged periods, at dosages that exceed the therapeutic range. Patients for whom I have been prescribed should be cautious about their use of alcohol because an additive effect may result.

Many of the most knowledgable people feel that I became the No. 1 prescribed medication in America because no other tranquilizer has been proven more effective. Or safer.

The FACT is they are right.

For a brief summary of product information on Valium (diazepam/Roche) ℞, please see the following page. Valium is available as 2-mg, 5-mg and 10-mg scored tablets.

FIGURE 9.11 (*continued*)

headlined "Examine Me" and "Feelings vs. Facts," had no real counterpart in prior prescription drug advertising.

Industry writer James Dickinson, describing Roche as "mellow as a bear trap when it needs to get around a government to defend a market," called the company "diabolically clever in wording ads in such a way that they came right up to, and maybe even onto, that national regulatory line that separates the permissible from the impermissible." Dickinson suggested that the FDA staff planned to limit its response to "jawboning" Roche into withdrawing the ads. Dr. Sidney Wolfe of Nader's Health

Feelings vs.

*Some people feel that I am misused and overused
and that I'm prescribed too often and for too many kinds
of problems.*

The FACT is that approximately eight million people,
or about 5 percent of the U.S. adult population, will use me
during the current year. By contrast, the national health
examination survey (1971-1975) found that 25 percent of
the U.S. adult population experiences moderate to severe
psychological distress. Additionally, studies of patient attitudes revealed that most patients have realistic views regarding the limitations of tranquilizers and a strong conservatism
about their use, as evidenced by a general tendency to
*de*crease intake over time. Finally, a six-year, large-scale,
carefully conducted national survey showed that the great
majority of physicians appropriately prescribe tranquilizers.

*Some people feel that patients being treated with anxiolytic
drugs are "weak," can't tolerate the anxieties of normal daily
living, and should be able to resolve their problems on their
own without the help of medication.*

The FACT is that while most people can withstand
normal, everyday anxieties, some people experience
excessive and persistent levels of anxiety due to personal
or clinical problems. An extensive national survey concluded
that Americans who do use tranquilizers have substantial

FIGURE 9.12

Resource Group, however, wanted much more. In a lengthy letter including
a substantial bibliography, Wolfe critiqued the ads almost sentence by
sentence and urged prompt and extensive FDA action.

Wolfe described the ads as "a desperate attempt by Roche Laboratories ... to stem the recent 45% decline in sales of Valium." The ads,
according to Wolfe, "suggest that Hoffmann-LaRoche, in order to regain
lost business, has become a white-collar dope pusher seeking new
business." Among Wolfe's suggestions to the FDA were to order Roche to
issue corrective ads; to advise physicians to write "no refill" on all

Facts

justification as evidenced by their high levels of anxiety. It was further noted that antianxiety drugs are not usually prescribed for trivial, transient emotional problems.

Some people feel afraid of me because of the stories they've heard about my being harmful and having the potential to produce physical dependence.

The FACT is that there are thousands of references in the medical literature documenting my efficacy and safety. Extensive and painstakingly thorough studies of toxicological data conclude that I am one of the safest types of psychotropic drugs available. However, I can produce dependence if patients do not follow their physicians' directions and take me for prolonged periods, at dosages that exceed the therapeutic range. Although infrequently seen, milder withdrawal symptoms have been reported following my abrupt discontinuance after being taken continuously, generally at higher therapeutic levels, for at least several months. Patients for whom I have been prescribed should be cautious about their use of alcohol because an additive effect may result.

— ADDED

Many of the most knowledgeable people feel that I became the No. 1 prescribed medication in America because no other tranquilizer has been proven more effective. Or safer.

The FACT is they are right.

For a brief summary of product information on Valium (diazepam/Roche)℞, please see the following page. Valium is available as 2-mg, 5-mg and 10-mg scored tablets.

FIGURE 9.12 (*continued*)

prescriptions for Valium and similar drugs; and to subject future ads to closer scrutiny.

The FDA did, in fact, require Roche to modify the ads. (The original and modified versions are shown as Figures 9.10 to 9.12.) But FDA Deputy Commissioner Mark Novitch noted that the FDA rejected the Wolfe proposals, stating that the ads, as changed, did not misrepresent the benefits and risks of Valium, "except for the section dealing with dependency."

Dr. Richard Dorsey, a frequent observer of public policy issues relating to psychiatry, reviewed in 1978 the then-pending Drug Regulation Reform Act of 1978 in the context of several FDA problems. Dorsey expressed concern about the level of science in the drug-regulating process, noting that the FDA Division of Neuropharmacological Drug Products was not, and had not been for some time, headed by a psychiatrist. Further, he stated, "The nature of regulation, with its emphasis on reviewing the word of others, adversary relationship with various groups, and vulnerability to political and legal considerations, rarely appeals to outstanding scientists."

Dorsey's concern about the level of science at the FDA became evident in his discussion of the proposed (under the 1978 bill) requirement that all drug research in humans, not just that of the drug companies, be conducted under FDA control. Dorsey (1978) wrote, "In addition to the obvious threat to academic freedom, this provision would have the bizarre result of requiring the most distinguished clinical investigators in the country to seek the approval of obscure FDA staffers whose principal qualification to act as arbiters of research consists of desks flanked by an American flag."

Dorsey had some critical comments about official drug labeling, noting that it constitutes a major source of prescribing information. His concerns included the possibility that local courts "may mistake labeling for a definitive scientific treatise rather than a regulatory document and give it undue weighting in defining a standard of practice in professional liability cases." Thus, according to Dorsey, "even the physician who has had considerable experience with a drug may be inclined to conform to the recommendations of the package insert in prescribing rather than rely on his or her own professional judgment."

Dorsey's problems with labeling went further. He noted that it is "intentionally biased in a strongly conservative direction" and, because it is so expensive to change it, is "at least as often obsolescent as authoritative." As an example, he cited Valium labeling, which warned against its use with epileptic patients at a time when it was recognized as the drug of choice for status epilepticus.

In 1980, Roche conducted a six-month trial of its own in an effort to determine consumer response to printed information dispensed with the prescription. The Roche patient information sheet (reprinted in part here) provides a broad range of data. Interesting comparisons may be drawn between the Roche presentation and official FDA labeling for MD consumption.

Roche Patient Labeling (indications)	FDA Physician Labeling
Valium is prescribed mainly to provide relief of: Anxiety and tension alone	Valium is indicated for the management of patients

(often experienced as difficulty sleeping, nervousness, and apprehension) or anxiety and tension when associated with other medical problems (for example, heart or stomach conditions). with certain anxiety disorders or anxiety associated with physical illness (e.g., acute myocardial infarction). [Valium] may also be indicated for the short-term relief of the symptoms of anxiety associated with significant transient situational disturbances. Mild anxiety or tension associated with the stress of everyday life usually does not require treatment with an anxiolytic.

The Roche organization was also disturbed by the article on Valium that appeared in *FDA Consumer* (Anon. 1980b). The article was distributed by Supermarket Communications, Inc., an FDA contrator, along with a poster that said "Valium?" The FDA agreed that use of the poster was both unauthorized and inappropriate, and both parties agreed to the publication of a letter stating this in *FDA Consumer*.

"SCHEDULING" THE MINOR TRANQUILIZERS

In July 1975, the benzodiazepines and meprobamate were officially added to the "Schedule IV" category of the Drug Enforcement Administration. This meant controls on refills, special record-keeping requirements for pharmacists, and, perhaps most importantly, an official statement that the drugs had abuse potential. The schedule had been a long time in coming.

In late 1965, both Librium and Valium had been recommended for scheduling by an advisory committee of the FDA. A long series of hearings followed both by the FDA and by the Bureau of Narcotics and Dangerous Drugs, which had taken over some of the regulatory responsibilities of the FDA. The tranquilizers essentially lost the battle in both sets of hearings, but escaped the controls again until Congress in 1970 included them in new legislation. (The manufacturers succeeded partially here, preventing inclusion of the minor tranquilizers in a category with barbiturates.)

Roche now exercised the right to petition for review by the U. S. Court of Appeals. The court, in March 1973, ruled that while the government had proved its case, Roche had been denied due process. For whatever reasons, Roche decided nevertheless (in August 1973) to submit to the controls. It still required two years to put the regulations into effect.

Falco (1980) describes the efforts of Roche to avoid scheduling of Librium and Valium as "the best known struggle between industry and the regulatory agencies over the imposition of controls."

> Through a series of complicated and costly legal maneuvers, Roche Labs succeeded in keeping its two tranquilizers free from government control for nearly ten years, until July 1975, despite the fact that the drugs were widely misused and were shown to produce physical dependence after chronic, high dose use. A primary reason for Roche's resistance to controls was the potential loss of sales. They estimated the sales loss would be between $10 and $20 million a year.

In fact, a decline in sales of minor tranquilizers had begun in 1973 (see Chapter 4). Crosby et al. (1978) analyzed the presumed effects of scheduling several drugs including diazepam. They found little effect on average prescription size in the year of or the year following schedule imposition.

MEDICAID AND THE MINOR TRANQUILIZERS

There are many fundamental questions concerning governmental limitation of its provision of health services that have not yet been answered. Drug formularies are an excellent example, specifically, the coverage of minor tranquilizers under Medicaid programs. Selection of the particular situation for discussion allows consideration of several facets of the right to health care.

Basic to the topic is the feeling held, rightly or wrongly, by thousands of people that the minor tranquilizers, if not actually happiness pills, do at least provide mitigation in situations causing considerable and often nonspecific unhappiness. In some ways, this puts the minor tranquilizers in a class by themselves, since they are often used to treat not easily defined symptoms such as high blood pressure or streptococcal infection, but rather, what some observers including FDA officials, have called "the problems of everyday living." Is payment for such drug use appropriate when it comes from the public coffers? In some states, the answer is "yes," in others, "no."

A review of drug coverage under Medicaid in several states reveals considerable variation with regard to the minor tranquilizers. In a few states, they are simply not covered—as a class. In a few others, only certain of these drugs are covered or are covered only for certain diagnoses or on special written request by the prescribing physician. As nearly as we can determine, such drugs are paid for in all states if such payment is part of the patient's hospital bill.

There is little or no evidence that restrictions on payment for minor tranquilizers are based on anything other than economic or perhaps even moral considerations.

Several states have deleted from or failed ever to include on their Medicaid formulary all or some of the minor tranquilizers. One of these was South Carolina, which deleted hydroxyzine and the benzodiazepines in July 1970 to "save money." Keeler and McCurdy (1975) studied the South Carolina situation using 12 months of Medicaid data equally divided before and after the formulary deletion. They concluded that there was no substitution of drugs still available for about two-thirds of the deleted minor tranquilizers. Following some rather shaky logic, they concluded that sedative barbiturates, filings for which increased, accounted for about 9 percent, hypnotics for 6.4 percent, phenothiazines for 15.4 percent, and tricyclic antidepressants for about 5 percent. The authors apparently did not consider the possibility that patients purchased prescriptions for the minor tranquilizers with their own funds.

Keeler and McCurdy were encouraged by their findings, which they interpreted to mean that physicians are cautious in prescribing sedatives, barbiturates, phenothizines, and tricyclic drugs. In fact, these drug classes increased by 15.4, 19.8, 29.9, and 3.2 percent, respectively—substantial increases in the use of drugs that are not, according to package inserts, interchangeable with the minor tranquilizers.

In discussing the deletion of the benzodiazepines from the South Carolina Medicaid formulary, Keeler and McCurdy argued that "the prevention of unnecessary discomfort is as much a part of medical paractice as is the prolongation of life, but it is not so dramatic." While it is true that relief of discomfort is a part of medical practice, it is not at all clear whether it is an expected component of publicly funded drug programs— by either the payer or the beneficiary. Certainly, coverage of such drugs is counter to the posture of pharmacological Calvinism discussed elsewhere.

In 1974, the state of Washington severely restricted the use of the minor tranquilizers in the Medicaid program. (Meprobamate was exempted from the restrictions.) Logerfo (1974) studied psychotropic drug use following these changes. He found no significant change in the utilization rates of other psychotropic drug use following deletion of the benzodiazepines, and similarly no statistically significant change in drug overdose cases by number, although the severity of cases involving drugs remaining on the formulary was greater.

With appropriate qualifications, Logerfo concluded that the total number of prescriptions for antianxiety agents "dropped dramatically" following formulary restrictions. If the drugs are at all necessary and effective, he wondered, was not the effect "to markedly reduce equity of access to relatively safe drugs which might relieve anxiety for many Medicaid recipients?" He noted that "this implies a double standard in our society with respect to why may receive these drugs."

In 1976–77, the Georgia Medicaid program also saw legal action. In a class action suit, an injunction was sought to prevent adoption of a "Controlled Medical Assisstance Drug List," in effect, a limited formulary. Although not aimed specifically at the minor tranquilizers, Librium and Valium would have been among the most popular drugs deleted.

The case turned on the issue of whether, following the adoption of the restrictive list, the Georgia Medicaid drug program would be "sufficient in amount, duration, and scope to reasonably achieve their purpose" as required by federal regulations.

Judge Rubard Freeman, granting the injunction, noted that the relevant statute was not entirely clear. Citing other cases and Title XIX, Freeman pointed out that the law "expressly recognizes financial matters as relevant considerations in fashioning Medicaid programs," but went on to observe that "in providing such services the discretion of the state is not unbridled." He concluded that the potential harm to the beneficiaries outweighed the recognized harm to the Medicaid program.

In 1978, the Pennsylvania Medical Society and the Pennsylvania Welfare Rights Organization joined forces in litigation against the State Department of Public Welfare (Bowers v. Colautti, civ. no. 3344, E. D. Pa. 1978). The issue was coverage of benzodiazepines under Medicaid.

On October 6, 1978, the Pennsylvania Pharmaceutical Association joined a number of other parties in filing suit against a number of officials of the Pennsylvania Department of Public Welfare (DPW). The issue was the impact of regulations that the department put into effect on October 1, which would deny payment by the state to pharmacists for certain drugs when they are prescribed for Medicaid recipients.

On May 6, 1978, the DPW gave notice of a proposed amendment to the regulations authorizing reimbursement for prescribed drugs. The proposed amendment made noncompensable all benzodiazepines except flurazepam, diazepam injection, and chlordiazepoxide. The noncompensable drugs were diazepam tablets, oxazepam, clonazepam, chlorazepate dipotassium, chlorazepate monopotassium, lorazepam, and prazepam. One September 23, 1978 (8 Pa. Bull 2634-2635), the department adopted the proposed regulations making all benzodiazepines noncompensable except the exempt drugs. The notice adopting the regulation stated:

> Numerous comments were recieved, all of which objected to the limitations on payment for benzodiazepines. Since medical evidence indicates that chlordiazepoxide is clinically equivalent to and may be

safely substituted for the more expensive brand name drugs, the proposed regulations are being adopted without modification.

The DPW intended that chlordizepoxide be substituted for the benzodiazepines made noncompensable by the challenged regulation. This was designed as an economy measure.

The basic complaint in the suit was that in totally prohibiting Medicaid reimbursement for the affected drugs, regardless of each Medicaid recipient's condition and medical necessity, the DPW's regulations deprived such recipients of equal protection under the law and of due process of law and conflict with the provisions of the applicable federal statute as well as Pennsylvania statutes and the department's own regulations. The arguments were as follows:

First, by promulgating and enforcing this regulation, the DPW caused Medicaid recipients who needed the affected drugs for proper medical treatment of their conditions to be deprived of their rights secured to them in the Medicaid legislation, in violation of the Equal Protection Clause of the Fourteenth Amendment to the U.S. Constitution.

Second, the regulation presumed, without any rational basis, the use of benzodiazepines, except for exempt drugs, is not medically necessary for the proper treatment of any person eligible for medical assistance. This violated (it was alleged) the due process clause of the Fourteenth Amendment to the U.S. Constitution.

Third, the regulation conflicted with federal Medicaid legislation in that it denied benefits to a class of medically needy persons on grounds unrelated to medical necessity, in violation of the supremacy clause of the U.S. Constitution.

Fourth, the regulation permitted some recipients of medical assistance to obtain medically necessary drugs for their health, while it denied medically necessary drugs to others. This violated state law, which requires that medical assistance services be administered uniformly.

Plaintiffs sought declaration that the regulation was invalid and unlawful and requested that the court enjoin the defendants from implementing or enforcing the regulation.

The DPW ultimately chose not to fight the suit and rather issued regulations (acceptable to the plaintiffs) that had as their intent the use of chlordizepoxide rather than other benzodiazepines. Physicians were "encouraged to do so in two ways. First, if the patient had a neurological disorder from a published list (epilepsy, spasticity due to central nervous system disease, dystonia, familial or essential tremor, "stiff-man" syndrome), a prescription for that diagnosis was required to be written if a benzodiazepine other than chlordizepoxide was to be dispensed. For other diagnoses, the physician was required to attach to the prescription a handwritten note listing the diagnosis and explaining why chlordiazepoxide was not acceptable as treatment. When chlordiazepoxide was prescribed generically, it was to be compensable, according to the proposed new rules, "for any medical condition."

In May 1979, Sidney Wolfe and Benjamin Gordon of Ralph Nader's Health Research Group recommended that the federal government not make further funds available for purchase of, inter alia, "anti-anxiety drugs (minor and major tranquilizers) except with prior authorization and when used for specific, approved indication" (Anon. 1979). Their view was that "the ordinary frustrations and tensions of daily living . . . are not really medical problems. Public Citizen's Health Research Group believes it is not appropriate for the taxpayers to finance the use of drugs for this purpose." No federal action ensued, however.

CONCLUSION

It should be apparent from the materials in this chapter that the minor tranquilizers caught and held the attention of legislators and regulators. As has so often been the case with these drugs, the results of this attention were equivocal and sometimes conflicting.

The courts, too, have been involved.

The turf of mental illness has been contested between law and medicine. In one well-known case (Rouse v. Cameron), the issue was whether the patient could be held in the hospital without an ongoing program of treatment. The court, apparently unsatisfied with less than specific answers concerning the antisocial behavior of the patient, finally declared (Ladimer 1975):

> I am not going to keep anybody deprived of his liberty on adjectives and generalities, it has got to be verbs and nouns, something that a person does or says that differentiates him from normal people and makes him dangerous. . . . Liberty is too precious to leave it merely to the opinions of psychiatrists. . . . Matters like these, in the ultimate analysis, *are for the court to determine.* [emphasis added]

An interesting service to the legal profession was described in the July 1980 issue of *Trial*. In the article devoted to problems with Valium, attorney Jonathan Zackey (1980) described the file system of the American Trial Lawyers Association (ATLA) Products Liability—Medical Malpractice Exchange. He noted the large number of inquiries received relative to the involvement of Valium in stillbirths and birth defects, and stated:

While legislative bodies and the FDA have examined this problem, the need still exists for the plaintiffs bar to cooperate in protecting the public from the overprescription of Valium. ATLA member attorneys handling diazepam cases are urged to contact the ATLA Exchange for cases, medical secondary references, and a list of other plantiff attorneys handling cases involving this drug.

Finally, Chauncey Leake (1970) was concerned about the growing pile of regulatory red tape—perhaps it causes anxiety.

There are minor psychiatric overtones to all of this [regulation]. Those who become involved, either from the standpoint of the development of new drugs or from the standpoint of regulating this development tend to become neurotic. Those who are interested in developing the new drugs tend to feel that they are being harassed and interfered with by the authoritarians who operate within the regulations. Those who are in authority tend to display it.

The enormous attention generated by these drugs in the sociolegal agencies confirms their existence as social facts. The struggles and relatively few final decisions resulting from this attention similarly confirm the existence of the cultural lag referred to in Chapter 1.

10

EPILOGUE

> "I always believe in six impossible things
> before breakfast."
>
> The Red Queen
> *Alice in Wonderland*

John Morgan (1980) has lucidly summarized some of the issues that have affected and continued to affect the minor tranquilizers.

> There is still much wrong with American prescribing habits. Some of what is wrong relates to our inability to view and to analyze the social context of drug use without recourse to the clinical ruse. Other problems include timidity, underprescribing, a costly Puritanical approach to needed therapy, and, in some instances (and only some), overprescribing.

In this brief epilogue, we will present a few developments that have occurred or seem about to occur at the close of a remarkable quarter-century.

ROOTS

New discoveries continue. Two important discoveries have helped in elucidating the mechanism of action of the benzodiazepines.

One such discovery was that Valium may enhance the actions of a neurotransmitter called γ-aminobutyric acid (GABA), which itself is an inhibitory neurotransmitter. That is, instead of promoting the flow of the nerve impulse across the synapse, Valium helps this decrease in flow, thus generally decreasing the nervous activity in the brain.

In Janury 1981, an entire issue of *Psychiatric Annals* was given over to the diagnosis and pharmacological management of anxiety disorders. Among the more intriguing discussions in this issue was the discovery that nerve cells in humans and animals possess "receptors" for benzodiazepine. The correlations cited between the binding site of the benzodiazepine and its therapeutic potency in humans suggest that the sites may mediate the pharmacological action of these drugs.

The significance of the findings just described goes well beyond a better understanding of the action of these drugs, for the presence of high-affinity binding sites in the brain suggests the existence of one or more endogenous compounds that act on the benzodiazepine receptor. Thus, the body may produce its own "Librium" or "Valium." Scientists, of course, are actively seeking to find and characterize any such endogenous compound. At the time of this article, some eight candidates had been suggested, but none could be unequivocally designated as endogenous benzodiazepine. (Interestingly, caffeine can bind to the receptor.)

The discovery of the benzodiazepine receptors in the human brain may contribute to our understanding of the mode of action of benzodiazepines and may eventually lead to the identification of a naturally occurring anxiety or antianxiety compound produced within the human brain that may play an important role in mediating behavioral symptoms of anxiety. (Note that it is generally assumed that treatment with an endogenous substance is far more acceptable than with a synthetic. This is one of the reasons for the excitement over the endorphins.)

As important as finding antianxiety agents is a better understanding of anxiety itself. A step in that direction is the discovery that certain compounds can produce anxietylike states in humans. These include piperoxan, lactate, and yohimbine. It also appears that one of the brain structures, the nucleus locus ceruleus, may mediate anxiety.

Bunney (1981) views all of these lines of research with considerable optimism: "Thus for the first time in many years, advances on several fronts have provided reason to hope that new understanding of the causes, prevention and treatment of anxiety will be forthcoming."

Heinz Lehmann (1977) has postulated the future of psychotropic drugs and offered the following predictions regarding anxiolytic drugs of the future:

- They will be truly specific.
- They will have built-in cutoff mechanisms based on negative feedback (in the same way that aspirin will not produce hypothermia).
- They will not produce increased conflict behavior.

- They will not produce or create physical or psychological dependence or tolerance.
- Toxicity will be minimal and there will be no synergism with other depressants.
- They will be safely prescribed even in early pregnancy.

Perhaps more important is the possibility of prevention. Mandershied (1976) suggested a future with a preventive orientation to mental problems. Included would be "brief classes in coping with stress and in interpersonal relations" as a part of general education at all levels. Also, greater attention would be given to delivering preventive mental health services at "critical points in the life cycle—adolescence, career beginnings, marriage, first child, etc."

UTILIZATION AND PRESCRIBING

In early 1983, the National Center for Health Statistics released results of its 1981 National Ambulatory Medical Care Survey (Koch 1983). These data showed that the class Tranquilizers, Sedatives, and Hypnotics represented 4.23 percent of all drug mentions, a slight decline over the previous year. In stark contrast to other data and earlier years, only three minor tranquilizer generic substances ranked in the top 100 most frequently used in office practice. The drugs and their ranks were

Diazepam—32
Chlordiazepoxide—60
Hydroxyzine—80

More detailed data, published later the same year, showed the benzodiazepines to account for 46.5 percent of all psychotropic drug mentions for the years 1980 and 1981. Of the top 25 psychotropic drugs, Valium continued to be the leader with 15.8 percent of all psychotropic prescriptions. Other minor tranquilizers with ranks (percentage) were

Tranxene	4(4.6)
Atarax	6(4.0)
Atiuan	8(3.5)
Librium	9(3.7)
Vistaril	14(2.2)
Meprobamate	15(2.1)
Centrax	22(1.4)
Serax	24(1.2)

Although the National Ambulatory Medical Care Survey data combine antianxiety agents, sedatives, and hypnotics into a single class, some of the findings concerning that class are worth attention. With regard to diagnosis, for example, this class of drugs demonstrated higher use rates than other psychotropics for the following diagnostic categories:

- Symptoms, signs, and ill-defined conditions
- Diseases of the circulatory system
- Diseases of the digestive system
- Diseases of the musculoskeletal system

Overall psychotropic drug use was higher among women than among men. This difference did not occur, however, until later years of age. Women in the 45- to 64-year age groups had a use rate one-third again as high as did men, and 60 percent more in the age category 65 and over.

Physicians in general practice and internal medicine accounted for two-thirds of all prescriptions for drugs in the class containing the antianxiety agents. Also interesting was the fact that physicians prescribed antianxiety agents for new patients at only half the rate as for old patients. The latter finding suggests a relatively conservative approach to therapy with the drugs.

THE ROAD FROM MILTOWN

Lay coverage of the minor tranquilizers continued, often in book form. *Stopping Valium* reached a second, revised edition in 1983. When Nader's Public Citizen Health Research Group published (Bargmann et al. 1982) the first edition, Roche brought suit charging trademark infringement. The company complained that "misuse of the Valium trademark as a generic term in reference to an entire group of drug products" should be stopped by an injunction against further publication and distribution of the book. Sydney Wolfe cited a disclaimer in the book's introduction that stated: "For the sake of simplicity, this book often refers to the entire group of the benzodiazepine family as Valium." The real reason for the Roche objection, according to Wolfe, was the content of the book that, he said, informs the public "about the addictive properties and other dangers of Valium" (*PMA Newsletter* 1982b).

Also in 1982, Paramount Pictures released *I'm Dancing as Fast as I Can*, a film based on the autobiography of Barbara Gordon. The film depicted Valium as the source of Gordon's psychological problems. Roche responded with a press release calling the film a demonstration of "blatant misuse" of the drug. Included in the release was the statement: "Perhaps the most cogent statement in the film is when Gordon complains that her problems are due to Valium and that is the reason she is in a mental institution. Her psychologist responds: 'I think you might have been here a lot sooner without it.'"

TELLING THE DOCTOR

Roche, still the leader in the field, was, in the early 1980s, providing prescribing guidelines through their advertising. They are reproduced here as offered by Dr. Bruce Medd, Roche's director of professional services.

GENERAL GUIDELINES FOR THE PRESCRIBING AND APPROPRIATE USE OF MINOR TRANQUILIZERS

- Individualize dosage for maximal beneficial effect.
- Prescribe no greater quantity than is needed until the next checkup period; schedule frequent, periodic checkups to monitor results of therapy.
- Establish treatment goals and discontinue medication when these have been met.
- Avoid prescribing for suicidal or dependency-prone individuals whose histories indicate an inability to handle any or all psychoactive substances including alcohol.
- Avoid undesirable interactions or development of drug misuse by evaluating patient's history regarding pattern of alcohol or drug consumption or use of nonprescription medication before prescribing minor tranquilizers.
- Caution patients against engaging in hazardous occupations requiring complete mental alertness such as operating machinery or driving.
- Counsel patients as to the proper use of the medication, such as following label directions, proper storage, and disposition of unused or old medication.
- Caution patients against giving medication to others.
- Avoid abrupt discontinuances of extended therapy and taper dosage in a gradual fashion.

Perhaps the most startling development of the advertising front was the dissertation of a doctoral student, John Mackowiak, at the University of North Carolina School of Pharmacy. Using IMS data and sophisticated statistical techniques, Mackowiak (1983) concluded that neither detailing nor journal advertising had any significant effect on the prescribing of benzodiazepines as a class or in influencing physicians to prescribe one of the drugs in preference to another. Given the strident criticism accorded pharmaceutical promotion of the minor tranquilizers, these findings are surprising indeed.

Mackowiak noted appropriately that his results may well have been affected by the fact that the benzodiazepines lie in the "mature" stage of the life cycle of a drug class described elsewhere in this text. Thus, a similar study conducted in the early 1960s would seem likely to have yielded different results. Nevertheless, Mackowiak's study, even with necessary qualifications, indicates that present promotion may be having minimal effects on prescribing and may be a comparative waste of someone's money.

REGULATION

In July 1981, the FDA submitted to the World Health Organization's Scientific Advisory Board an extensive packet of information on the benzodiazepine class of drugs. The impetus for the submission was concern about the abuse liability of this class of drugs, which had become the most widely used drug class in history.

The FDA action was significant as a historical marker at the end of the first quarter-century of experience with a group of drugs that had come to be known as the "minor tranquilizers" and that had begun with the marketing of meprobamate in 1955. The FDA report, the deliberations that preceded it, and the conclusions that it reached—and failed to reach—offer, in many ways, a microcosm of the struggles that medicine and society have had in evaluating these fascinating drugs.

In May 1981, the FDA Bureau of Drugs Drug Abuse Advisory Committee held a two-day open meeting to discuss the benzodiazepines. The purpose was "an assessment of the abuse liability" of the class of products pursuant to a recommendation to the World Health Organization.

Hoffmann-LaRoche submitted eight volumes of information to the committee. The Roche position, as summarized by Director of Scientific and Public Information Robert Jones, included eight points:

1. Widespread concern about benzodiazepine dependence is based largely on anecdotal material rather than sound scientific evidence.
2. Much of the concern about the misuse potential of the benzodiazepines has been exaggerated.

3. Dependence on benzodiazepines occurs rarely under conditions of clinical use, and then only after prolonged administration at high doses.
4. Withdrawal symptoms may follow abrupt discontinuation of any benzodiazepine and therefore gradual discontinuation is appropriate.
5. Prevalence of tranquilizer use is consistent and logical based on worldwide morbidity data.
6. The American public is unreasonably concerned and confused about benefit/risk aspects of prescription tranquilizer use.
7. Data do not support allegations that benzodiazepines are used for trivial problems of everyday life.
8. Patients do not generally tend to increase diazepam dosage over time.

Dr. David Smith, a member of the committee and a student of drug abuse, summarized some of the data on abuse potential. He described benzodiazepine dependence as "an extremely complicated dynamic process," suggesting that misinformation generated by the drug industry and by the lay press was a contributing factor. He objected to a statement made earlier by Dr. Sidney Wolfe that the consumer was a "pure victim." Rather, he stated, the physician is often manipulated by the patient.

Dr. Carl Chambers of Ohio University addressed the risk to the public health. His opinion was that there was considerable misuse, but of a self-medication rather than a pleasure-seeking nature. Both physical and especially psychological dependence were viewed as problems and the environment surrounding the benzodiazepines was characterized as one of "seduction"—helped by the industry, neither physicians, pharmacists, nor patients viewed benzodiazepines as "drugs." Based on his own research, Chambers concluded that 10–15 percent of physicians liberally prescribed the drugs and 10–15 percent of consumers misused them in some way. He did not perceive the drugs to be a major public health hazard.

Committee member Sidney Cohen described his three-part "law of the new miracle drug" (see Chapter 1) at this conference, and Dr. Karl Rickels, in other documents submitted for study, concluded that (1) Psychotropic drugs are conservatively used and possibly even underused at times; (2) Patient attitudes express doubts concerning the morality of drug use and are associated with traditional stoic values; (3) Little support is provided for a "self-indulgent" consumer interpretation of drug use; (4) The majority of physicians are conservative and rather astute in their psychotropic drug-prescribing habits. More research was needed, however. Rickels suggested the following studies:

- Addiction potential, including patient characteristics
- Indications for long-term benzodiazepine treatment
- The phenomena of drug withdrawal
- Sociological studies of benzodiazepine use
- Effects on memory, cognition, performance
- Role in physical illness
- Use in the elderly

The U. S. Department of Health and Human Services recommended Schedule IV status for 26 benzodiazepines by the World Health Organization. In February 1983, however, the U.N. Commission on Narcotic Drugs voted against that action, calling instead for another review.

WHERE ARE WE NOW?

Marks (1981) has published a number of papers arguing that the dependence risk of the benzodiazepines is low, given their wide use. As noted in Chapter 1, he too suggests that the benzodiazepines may be about to reach the "rational therapeutic use point."

In March 1984, the Division of Drug Experience of the FDA published utilization statistics showing that nearly one of every ten prescriptions contained either hydrochlorothiazide or codeine (Baum et al. 1984). No outcry of over use ensued. Nor was much attention given to the third-ranking drug category, "combination oral contraceptives." Yet the minor tranquilizers, and the benzodiazepines in particular, have, almost from the beginning, been viewed with sincere concern whenever they led, or were among the leaders of, drug use statistics.

Our struggles to deal with the role of the minor tranquilizers, very real in its own right, is also part of several other social concerns including the future role of the physician. Many of the issues that these drugs have caused to surface have yet to be resolved. Each of us will be involved in that resolution.

Mary Davis (1977) has described the kind of problem we face:

The role of the physician, according to Webster, is to "treat diseases"; a physician is one "skilled in the art of healing." This seems a clear enough statement, one which should occasion little controversy, and yet many people today are confused as to exactly what duties a physician is to perform. It is widely accepted that one's life style and environment may be etiological factors in diseases such as ulcers and hypertension (as well, of course, as many psychiatric diseases). Does it then become the physician's responsibility to modify the life style or environment of the patient? Each physician must, finally, answer this question for himself, deciding where lies the dividing line between medical practice and unwarranted interference in another's life. Society, however, has not yet drawn this line clearly; until it does so physicians and patients alike will continue to be confused regarding the physician's role.

It is an intentional oversimplification to describe the minor tranquilizers as drugs used to treat the symptoms of minor mental irregularity—not so different from a laxative, antacid, or cold tablet, except that they affect the mind. While certainly not innocuous, they are also not as dramatically dangerous as, for example, LSD. Yet we have dealt with these drugs in an emotional, sometimes irrational fashion. Kline (1971) said, "There seems to be a icebox built somewhere into our skulls which is the seat of cold logic and rational thought, and next to it is a hothouse of irrational, affect-based beliefs," and the two do not interact. Indeed, that seems often to have been the case with our views of the minor tranquilizers.

Well, we survived.

By luck, perhaps by growing sophistication in the field of mental health, and by other means, we may have reached a form of stability regarding this class of drugs as they now exist.

But what next?

Nearly 15 years ago, Kline (1971) suggested that the year 2000 would see drugs that, inter alia,

- Provide safe, short-acting intoxication
- Prolong or shorten memory
- Provoke or relieve guilt
- Control affect and aggression
- Shorten or extend experienced time.

These and other predictions were not idle futuristic exercises, but rather serious predictions of a knowledgeable scientist.

Surely it is time to review our performance with the comparatively simple drugs we have had for a quarter-century or more, to attempt to discovery how better to deal with those that are to come.

BIBLIOGRAPHY

Abbott, L., Freeman, R., and Froelich, R. L. 1983, "Psychiatric Diagnosing Rates of Family Practice Physicians," *Resident and Staff Physician*, 29:25–36.

Abroms, G., and Greenfield, N. 1972, "Drug Prescribing and the Mental Health Professions: A Proposal," *International Journal of Psychiatry*, 10:70–81.

Aden, G. 1978, "Forward." In *Principles of Psychopharmacology* (2nd ed.), edited by W. Clark and J. del Giudice. New York: Academic Press, pp. 7–8.

Altman, H. et al. 1972, "Patterns of Psychotropic Drug Prescription in Four Midwestern State Hospitals," *Current Therapeutic Research* 14:667–672.

America. 1958, "Tranquilizers and Ethics," October 11, p. 32.

American Mercury. 1960, "To Tranquilize or Not To Tranquilize," September, p. 153.

American Psychiatric Association. 1980, *Diagnostic and Statistical Manual for Mental Disorders*, (3rd ed.). Washington, D.C.

Annitto, W., and Kass, W. 1979, "Psychotherapy, Psychopharmacology, and the Illusion of Curing," *Bulletin of the Menninger Clinic*, 43:552–555.

Anon. 1981a, "Benzodiazepines," Rockville: Department of Health and Human Services, Processed.

Anon. 1981b, "Proposed Valium Ad Regulations Shot Down by FDA Topsiders," *Drug Store News*, 3:36.

Anon. 1981c, "Drug Utilization in the United States, 1980," Rockville: Food and Drug Administration.

Anon. 1980a, "Guidelines for Prescribing Controlled Substances," *DEA/Registrant Facts*, 6:1–2.

Anon. 1980b, "Overcoping with Valium," *FDA Consumer*, 13:21–23.

Anon. 1980c, "Teleflashes," *American Druggist*, 182:1.

Anon. 1979, "Medicaid Payment for 'Inferior' R_x Drugs." *F–D–C Reports*, 41:13.

Anon. 1974, "International Use of Tranquilizers," *British Medical Journal*, 2:300.

Anon. 1973. "Benzodiazepines: Use, Overuse, Misuse, Abuse?" *Lancet*, 297:1101–1102.

Anon. 1967, "Today's Drug Benzodiazepines," *British Medical Journal*, 2:36–38.

Anon. n.d., "Sixty Minutes Interview (Transcript)," Supplied by Roche Laboratories.

Appleton, W. 1967, "A Guide to the Use of Psychoactive Agents," *Diseases of the Nervous System*, 28:609–613.

Armstrong, D. 1980, "Madness and Coping," *Sociology of Health and Illness*, 2:296–316.

Asken, M. 1979, "Medical Psychology: Toward Definition, Clarification, and Organization," *Professional Psychology*, 10:66–73.

Avroutski, G. 1968, "The Vogue of the Pill (Tranquilizer That Is)," *Unesco Courier*, 21:20–23.

Ayd, F. 1980, "Social Issues: Misuse and Abuse," *Psychosomatics*, 21:21–26.

_____. 1975, "Oxazepam: An Overview," *Diseases of the Nervous System*, 36:14–16.

_____. 1970, "The Impact of Biological Psychiatry," In *Discoveries in Biological Psychiatry*, edited by B. Blackwell, pp. 230–243. Philadelphia: J. B. Lippincott.

_____. 1968, "Is Psychiatry in a Crisis Because of the Complications of Psychopharmaceuticals?" *Diseases of the Nervous System*, 29:23–25.

Azima, H. 1956a, "Drugs for the Mind," *Nation*, 183:56–59.

_____. 1956b, "Truth About the Tranquilizers," *Science Digest*, 40:71–74.

Balser, M. et al. 1977, "Use of Tranquilizing Drugs by a Middle-Aged Population in a West German City," *Journal of Health and Social Behavior*, 18:194–205.

Balter, M. 1975, "Coping with Illness: Choices, Alternatives and Consequences." In *Drug Development and Marketing*, edited by R. Helms, pp. 27–45. Washington, D.C.: American Enterprise Institute for Public Policy Research.

_____. 1973, "An Analysis of Psychotherapeutic Drug Consumption in the United States," Anglo-American Conference on Drug Abuse, Royal Society of Medicine, pp. 58–68.

Balter, M., and Levine, J. 1971, "Character and Extent of Psychotherapeutic Drug Usage in the United States," *Psychiatry I* (Excerpta Medica) 23:80–88.

_____. 1969, "The Nature and Extent of Psychotropic Drug Usage in the United States," *Psychopharmacology Bulletin*, 5:3–13.

Balter, M., et al. 1975, "Patterns of Prescribing and Use of Hypnotic Drugs in the United States." In *Sleep Disturbance and Hypnotic Drug Dependence*, edited by A. D. Clift, pp. 261–293. Amsterdam: Excepta Medica.

Balter, M., Levine, J., and Manheimer, D. 1974a, "Drug Use as Determined by Interviews," *New England Journal of Medicine*, 290:1491.

_____. 1974b, "Cross National Study of the Extent of Anti-Anxiety/Sedative Drug Use," *New England Journal of Medicine*, 290:769–774.

Bargmann, E., Wolfe, S.M., and Levin, J. 1982, *Stopping Valium*. Washington, D.C.: The Public Citizen Health Research Groups.

Barletta, M. 1978, "Psychotropic Drugs...An Update," *American Druggist*, 177:43–46.

Baron, S., and Fisher, S. 1952, "Use of Psychotropic Drug Prescriptions in a Prepaid Group Practice Plan," *Public Health Reports*, 77:871–882.

Barton, R., and Hurst, L. 1966, "Unnecessary Use of Tranquilizers in Elderly Patients," *British Psychiatric Journal*, 112:989–990.

Baum, C. et al. 1984, "Drug Use in the United States in 1981," *Journal of the American Medical Association*, 251:1293–1297.

Bellantuomo, C. et al. 1980, "Benzodiazepines: Clinical Pharmacology and Therapeutic Use," *Drugs*, 19:195.

Benedict, J. 1960, "Mind Control/The Ultimate Tyranny," *American Mercury*, 90:12–27.

Beig, R. 1971, "The Over-Medicated Woman," *McCalls*, 98:67.

———. 1956, "The Unhappy Facts About 'Happy Pills'," *Look*, 20:92.

Berger, F. 1978, "Introduction: The Aims and Achievements of Psychopharmacology." In *Principles of Psychopharmacology*, edited by W. Clark and J. del Giudice. New York: Academic Press, pp. 1–9.

———. 1970, "Anxiety and the Discovery of the Tranquilizers." In *Discoveries in Biological Psychiatry*, edited by F. Ayd and B. Blackwell. Philadelphia: J. B. Lippincott, pp. 1–9.

Berger, F. 1964, "The Tranquilizer Decade," *Journal of Neuropsychiatry*, 5:403–410.

Berger, P. 1978, "Medical Treatment of Mental Illness," *Science*, 200:974–981.

Bergman, V. et al. 1979, "Why Are Psychotropic Drugs Prescribed to Out-Patients?" *European Journal of Clinical Pharmacology*, 15:249–256.

Berland, T., 1961, "Quiet Pills Are No Short-Cut," *Today's Health*, 39:34, 68–69.

Bishop, J. 1979, "Age of Anxiety-Stress of American Life Is Increasingly Blamed for Emotional Turmoil," *Advertising Age*, 50:17.

Blackwell, B. 1975a, "Rational Drug Use in Psychiatry." In *Rational Pharmacology and the Right to Treatment*, edited by F. J. Ayd, pp. 187–199. Baltimore: Ayd Medical Communications.

———. 1975b, "Minor Tranquilizers: Use, Misuse or Overuse?" *Psychosomatics*, 16:28–31.

———. 1973a, "Psychotropic Drugs in Use Today," *Journal of the American Medical Association*, 225:1637–1641.

———. 1973b, "Tranquilizer Control," *Journal of the American Medical Association*, 223:798.

———. 1970, "The Process of Discovery." In *Discoveries in Biological Psychiatry*, edited by F. J. Ayd, pp. 11–27. Philadelphia: J. B. Lippincott.

(Blatnik) 1958, "False and Misleading Advertising (Prescription Tranquilizing Drugs)." Hearings before the (Senate) Subcommittee of the Committee on Government Operations, Washington, D.C.

Blau, S. 1978, "A Guide to the Use of Psychotropic Medication in Children and Adolescents," *Journal of Child Psychiatry*, 39:776–782.

Blough, D. 1958, "New Test for Tranquilizers," *Science*, 127:586–587.

Boe, S. 1971, "The Increasing Use of Prescription and Over-the-Counter Psychoactive Drugs by Adults in the United States," *Journal of Drug Issues*, 1:386–394.

Boethius, G., and Westerholm, B. 1977, "Purchases of Hypnotics, Sedatives and Minor Tranquilizers Among 2,566 Individuals in County of Jamtland, Sweden," *Acta Psychiatrica Scandinavia*, 56:147–159.

Bond, W. 1980, "The Clinical Use of Antianxiety Agents," *American Druggist*, 182:36–39.

_____. 1979, "The Clinical Use of Antidepressants," *American Druggist*, 179:35–39.

Borrus, J. 1955, "Study of Effect of Miltown on Psychiatric States," *Journal of the American Medical Association*, 152:1591 1598.

Brahen, L. 1973, "Housewife Drug Abuse," *Journal of Drug Education*, 13:13–24.

Branca, P. 1977. *The Medicine Show*. New York: Science History Publications.

Brands, A., and Towery, O. 1980, "Psychotropic Drugs—Approaches to Psychopharmacologic Drug Use," Division for Health and Human Services, pp. 3–71.

Braswell, H., and Williamson, J. 1979, "Assessing Depression Outcomes in Group Practice Clinics," *American Journal of Public Health*, 69:1281–1283.

Brockman, J., and D'Arcy, C. 1978, "Correlates of Attitudinal Social Distance Toward the Mentally Ill: A Review and a Re-Survey," *Social Psychiatry*, 13:69–77.

Brown, B., Regier, D., and Balter, M. 1977, "Key Interactions Among Psychiatric Disorders, Primary Care and the Use of Psychotropic Drugs," *Excerpta Medica*, pp. 1–16.

Bruhn, J. 1977–78, "When Does a Drug Become a Social Problem?" *Drug Forum*, 6:207–214.

Bunney, W. 1981, "Current Biologic Strategies for Anxiety," *Psychiatric Annals*, 11:11–15.

Burger, A. 1976. "History." In *Psychotherapeutic Drugs, Part I—Principles*, edited by E. Usdin, pp. 11–57. New York: Marcel Dekker.

Burney, L. 1958, "Once over Unsettling Facts About Tranquilizers," *Consumer Reports*, 23:4.

Business Week. 1960, "Tranquilizer Makers Put on Spot," February 6, p. 32.

Business Week. 1958, "Tranquil Pills Stir up Doctors," June 28, pp. 28, 30.

Business Week. 1956, "No Peace for Tranquilizers," September 1, p. 32.

Bylinsky, G. 1976, "Future Drugs That Will Be Lifesavers for the Industry Too," *Fortune*, 94:152–162.

Caldwell, A. 1978. "History of Psychopharmacology." In *Principles of Psychopharmacology*, edited by W. Clark and J. del Guidice. New York: Academic Press, pp. 9–41.

_____. 1970. *Origins of Psychopharmacology from CPZ to LSD*. Springfield: Charles C Thomas.

Callen, K., and Davis, D. 1978, "The General Practitioner: How Much Psychiatric Education?" *Psychosomatics*, 19:21–23.

Cant, G. 1976. "Valiumania," *New York Times*, February 1, pp. 34–54.

Carey, G., Gottesman, I., and Robins, E. 1980, "Prevalence Rates for the Neuroses:

Pitfalls in the Evaluation of Familiarity," *Psychological Medicine*, 10:437–443.

Carmody, J., Boyle, B., Butler, P., Douglas, P., and Dwyer, D. 1977, "Patterns of the Use of Benzodiazepines in Australia," *Medical Journal of Australia*, 2:666–668.

Chaiton, A. et al. 1976, "Patterns of Medical Drug Use—A Community Focus," *Canadian Medical Association Journal*, 114:33–37.

Chambers, C. 1972. "An Assessment of Drug Use in the General Population." In *Drug Use and Social Policy*, edited by J. Susman, pp. 50–61. New York: AMS Press.

Chapman, J. et al. 1966, "Relationships of Stress, Tranquilizers, and Serum Cholesterol Levels in a Sample Population Under Study for Coronary Heart Disease," *American Journal of Epidemiology*, 83:537–547.

Chapman, S. 1979, "Advertising and Psychotropic Drugs: The Place of Myth in Ideological Reproduction," *Social Science and Medicine*, 13A:751–764.

_____. 1976, "Psychotropic Drug Use in the Elderly," *Medical Journal of Australia*, 2:62–64.

Changing Times. 1962, "Drugs for the Mind," July, pp. 19–21.

Changing Times. 1956, "The Facts About Those Happy Pills," October, pp. 23–24.

Christian Century. 1956, "Happiness Pills Are No Answer," September 12, p. 1044.

Coates, D. "On the Edge of a Nervous Breakdown." Unpublished paper quoted in Cooperstock and Parnell (1982).

Cohen, I. 1970, "The Benzodiazepines." In *Discoveries in Biological Psychiatry*, edited by F. Ayd and B. Blackwell. Philadelphia: J. B. Lippincott, pp. 130–135.

Cohen, J., Gomez, E., and Hoell, N. 1976, "Diazepam and Phenobarbital in the Treatment of Anxiety: A Controlled Multicenter Study Using Physician and Patient Rating Scales," *Current Therapeutic Research*, 20:184–193.

Cole, S., and Lejeune, R. 1972, "Illness and Legitimation of Failure," *American Sociological Review*, 37:347–356.

Coleman, J., and Patrick, D. 1978, "Psychiatry and General Health Care," *American Journal of Public Health*, 68:451–457.

Coleman, L., and Solomon, T. 1976, "Big Brother Knows Best," *Psychology Today*, 10:85–88.

Colen, B. 1980a. "Valium—'Psychic Aspirin'—Abused as Tranquilizer." *Clarion Ledger*, February 10, p. G1.

_____. 1980b. "Chemist's Tenacity Led to Most Widely Prescribed Drug." *Clarion Ledger*, February 10, p. G3.

Committee on Public Health, New York Academy of Medicine. 1964, "Misuse of Valuable Therapeutic Agents: Barbiturates, Tranquilizers and Amphetamines," *Bulletin of New York Academy of Medicine*, 40:972–979.

"Competitive Problems in the Drug Industry Drug Testing." 1979, Summary and Analysis, (Senate) Select Committee on Small Business, Washington, D.C.

"Competitive Problems in the Drug Industry Psychotropic Drugs." 1979, Summary and Analysis, (Senate) Select Committee on Small Business, Washington, D.C.

Consumer Reports. 1971a, "More Drugs to Think Twice About," March, pp. 180–181.

Consumer Reports. 1971b, "Some Medicines You May Want to Avoid," February, pp. 114–117.

Consumer Reports. 1967, "Tranquilizers and Other Psychoactive Drugs—How Well Do They Work?" October, pp. 544–550.

Consumer Reports. 1955, "Wonder Drugs and Mental Disorders," August, pp. 386–389.

Cooley, D. 1956. "The New Drugs That Make You Feel Better." *Cosmopolitan,* September, pp. 24–27.

Cooperstock, R. 1978a. "Women and Psychotropic Drug Use." In *The Chemically Dependent Women,* edited by J. Dowsling and A. MacLennan. Toronto: Addiction Research Foundation, pp. 39–48.

———. 1978b, "Sex Differences in Psychotropic Drug Use," *Social Science and Medicine,* 12B:179–186.

Cooperstock, R., and Leonard, H. 1979, "Some Social Meanings of Tranquilizer Use," *Sociology of Health and Illness,* 1:331–347.

Cooperstock, R., and Parnell, P. 1982, "Research on Psychotropic Drug Use," *Social Science and Medicine,* 16:1179–1196.

Cornely, P. 1978, "Comments on Welfare Status, Illness and Subjective Health Definition," *American Journal of Public Health,* 68:870–871.

Coronet. 1957. "The Whole Story About Those Peace-of-Mind Pills," April, pp. 66–70.

Cousins, Norman 1984. "Unacceptable Pressures on the Physician," *Journal of the American Medical Association,* 252:351–352.

Cowen, D. 1960, "Those Pretty Little Pills," *Nation,* 190:335–338.

Craig, T., and Van Natta, P. 1978, "Current Medication Use and Symptoms of Depression in a General Population," *American Journal of Psychiatry,* 135:1036–1039.

Crosby, D., Burke, L., and Kennedy, J. 1978, "Drug Scheduling—What Effects?" Paper presented at the American Pharmaceutical Association Annual Meeting, Montreal.

Crout, J. (testimony). 1976, "Competitive Problems in the Drug Industry," Hearings before the Subcommittee on Monopoly of the Select Committee on Business, U.S. Senate, Part 30, May 24.

Cullen, W. 1798, *A Treatise of the Materia Medica.* Edinburgh: Elliott.

Cutler, N., and Heiser, J. 1978, "The Tricyclic Antidepressants," *Journal of the American Medical Association,* 240:2264–2266.

Cypress, B. 1978, "Office Visits to Psychiatrists: National Ambulatory Medical Care Survey, United States, 1975–76," Advance Data, U.S. Department Health and Human Services, August 25, pp. 1–8.

Davidson, J., Raft, D., and Lewis, B. 1975, "Psychotropic Drugs on General Medical and Surgical Wards of a Teaching Hospital," *Archives of General Psychiatry,* 32:507–511.

Davies, B. 1973, "Diagnosis and Treatment of Anxiety and Depression in General Practice," *Practical Therapeutics*, 6:389–399.

Davis, J. 1965, "Efficacy of Tranquilizing and Antidepressant Drugs," *Archives of General Psychiatry*, 13:552–572.

Davis, M. 1977, "Disease and Its Treatment," *Comprehensive Psychiatry*, 18:231.

Davis, W. 1960, "Doctors Need Tranquilizers," *Science News Letter*, 77:148.

Dean, R. 1971, "Comments on the Proceedings—6th Annual Institue on Man's Adjustment in a Complex Environment and Reaction to Turner," *Journal of Drug Issues*, 6:1.

DeKruif, P. 1961, "The First Tranquilizer," *Saturday Review*, 44:70–71.

del Giudice, J. 1978. "Clinical Use of Anxiolytic Drugs in Psychiatry." In *Principles of Psychopharmacology*, edited by W. Clark and J. del Giudice, pp. 561–572. New York: Academic Press.

Denber, H., Abroms, G., and Greenfield, N. 1972, "Drug Prescribing: Critical Evaluation (Author's Reply)," *International Journal of Psychiatry*, 10:90–93.

Deniker, P. 1966, *La Psychopharmacologie*. Paris: Presses Universitaires de France.

Dennis, P. 1979, "Monitoring of Psychotropic Drug Prescribing in General Practice," *British Medical Journal*, 2:1115–1116.

DeSilverio, R., Rickels, K., Raab, E., and Jameson, J. 1969, "Oxazepam and Meprobamate in Anxious Neurotic Outpatients," *Journal of Clinical Pharmacology*, 9:259–263.

Dickinson, J. 1981, "HRG Witnesses FDA's New Spirit," *Pharmaceutical Executive*, 1:16–17.

DiGiacomo, J., and Rosen, H. 1980, "Psychosomatic Disorders: Psychotropic Medications," *Psychosomatics*, 20:75–79.

DiMascio, A. 1975. "Innovative Drug Administration Regimens and the Economics of Mental Health Care." In *Rational Pharmacotherapy and the Right to Treatment*, edited by F. Ayd, pp. 118–130. Baltimore: Ayd Medical Communications.

DiMascio, A., and Goldberg, H. 1978, "Recognizing and Treating Anxiety," *Current Prescribing*, 10:17–26.

DiMascio, A. et al. 1979, "Psychopharmacological Screening Criteria Development Project," *Journal of the American Medical Association*, 241:1021–1031.

(Dingell) 1967, "Small Business Problems in the Drug Industry." Hearings before the (House) Subcommittee on Activities of Regulatory Agencies of the Select Committee on Small Business, Washington, D.C., Volumes 1 and 2.

Ditzion, B. 1971, "Psychotropic Drug Advertisements," *Annals of Internal Medicine*, 75:473–474.

Dodson, E. V. Parham, T. 1977, "Order-Controlled Medical Assistance Drug List," U.S. District Court, Northern District of Atlanta, Georgia.

Dohrenwend, D., and Dohrenwend, B. 1974, "Sex Differences and Psychiatric Disorders," Paper presented at the VIII Congress of Sociology, Toronto, August 19, 1974.

Donagan, A. 1978. "How Much Neurosis Should We Bear?" In *Mental Health:*

Philosophical Perspectives, edited by H. Engelhardt and S. Spicker. Boston: D. Reidel, pp. 41–43.

Dorsey, R. 1978, "The American Psychiatric Association and the Food and Drug Administration: An Analysis and Proposal for Action," *American Journal of Psychiatry*, 135:1049–1056.

———. 1975, "Peer Review of Psychotropic Drug Use." In *Rational Pharmacotherapy and the Right to Treatment*, edited by F. Ayd, pp. 176–186. Baltimore: Ayd Medical Communications.

Dorsey, R., Ayd, F., Cole, J., Klein, D., Simpson, G., and Tupin, J. 1979, "Psychological Screening Criteria Development Project," *Journal of the American Medical Association*, 241:1021.

Dowling, H. 1963, "How Do Practicing Physicians Use New Drugs?" *Journal of the American Medical Association*, 185:87–90.

Drossman, D. 1977–78, "Can the Primary Care Physician Be Better Trained in the Psycho-Social Dimensions of Patient Care?" *International Journal of Psychiatry in Medicine*, 8:169–184.

Dunlop, D. 1971, "The Use and Abuse of Psychotropic Drugs," *Scottish Medical Journal*, 16:345–349.

———. 1970, "Abuse of Drugs by the Public and by Doctors," *British Medical Journal*, 26:236–239.

Dunn, G. 1981, "The Diagnosis and Classification of Anxiety States," *Psychiatric Annals*, 11:6–10.

Eastwood, M., and Trevelyn, M. 1972, "Relationship Between Physical and Psychiatric Disorder," *Psychological Medicine*, 2:363–372.

Edelstein, E., Esac, M., and Stein, J. 1973, "How Antagonistic Can Doctor's Bias Be on Drug Effect?" *International Pharmacopsychiatry*, 8:37–59.

Elkes, J. 1978. "Epilogue and Foreglimpse." In *Principles of Psychopharmacology*, edited by W. Clark and J. del Giudice, pp. 741–743. New York: Academic Press.

Elliott, C., and Kintzler, C. 1973, "No Prescription Pads for Social Workers," *Clinical Social Work Journal*, 1:134–136.

Elliott, H. 1973, "Clinial Pharmacology," *Postgraduate Medicine*, 54:159–164.

Engelhardt, H., Jr. 1978. "Introduction." In *Mental Health: Philosophical Perspectives*, edited by H. Engelhardt and S. Spicker, pp. 4–6. Boston: D. Reidel.

Evans, W. 1971, "Why Don't They Believe Us Anymore? Or Hypocrisy, Social Change and Credibility," *Journal of Drug Issues*, 6:333–338.

Falco, M. 1980. "The Pharmaceutical Industry and Drug Use and Misuse." In *The Community's Response to Drug Use*, edited by S. Einstein, pp. 317–338. New York: Pergamon Press.

Farm Journal. 1958a, "Tranquilizer in Feed OK'd for Beef," October, p. 54.

Farm Journal. 1958b, "Latest on Tranquilizers," January, p. 43.

Farm Journal. 1957, "Now It's Tranquilizers for Hens," September, p. 32.

FDC Reports. 1980a, "Roche Meeting with FDA Com. Goyan on 'Over Medication'," July 21, p. 3.

FDC Reports. 1980b, "Roche Valium Patient Labeling Includes Use for Anxiety and Tension Along," February 4, pp. 7–8.

FDC Reports. 1979a, "Benzodiazepine Label Revision—To Deplete 'Stress' Indications," December 3, pp. I, G1.

FDC Reports. 1979b, "Upjohn Benzodiazepine Xanax Okay for Symptomatic Relief," October 22, pp. 8–9.

FDC Reports. 1979c, "Benzodiazepine MD Label Changes: Stress and Stressful Situation Indications Are Being Revived by FDA, Crout Tells Kennedy," September 17, pp. 1–8.

Federspiel, C., Ray, W., and Schaffner, W. 1980, "A Study of Antipsychotic Drug Use in Nursing Homes: Epidemiologic Evidence Suggesting Misuse," *American Journal of Public Health*, 70:485–491.

Feinbloom, R. 1971a, "To Open Debate on Tranquilizers," *New England Journal of Medicine*, 284:790–791.

_____. 1971b, (Testimony) "Advertising of Proprietary Medicines." Hearings before the Subcommittee on Monopoly of the Select Committee on Small Business, U.S. Senate, Part 2, p. 503.

Fejer, D., and Smart, R. 1973, "The Use of Psychoactive Drugs by Adults," *Canadian Psychiatric Association Journal*, 18:313–319.

Finkle, B., McCloskey, K., and Goodman, L. 1979, "Diazepam and Drug Associated Deaths," *Journal of the American Medical Association*, 242:429–434.

Fisher, J. 1976, "Complications of Psychoactive Drugs as Seen by Family Practitioners," *Psychiatric Forum*, 5:8–23.

Fleischman, M. 1968, "Will the Real Third Revolution Please Stand Up?" *American Journal of Psychiatry*, 124:146–148.

Fortune. 1963, "The Untranquilized Drug Makers," December, pp. 124–129, 202–204, 209.

(Fountain) 1969, "Regulation of Prescription Drug Advertising." Thirty-Ninth Report of the (House) Committee on Government Operations, Washington, D.C.

Freedman, D. 1979, "Will the Real Doctor Please Stand Up?" *Archives of General Psychiatry*, 36:1399–1400.

Friedson, E. 1970. *Profession of Medicine.* New York: Dodd, Mead.

Fritz, G., Collins, G., and Biernoff, M. 1979, "The Use of Minor Tranquilizers in a Community Mental Health Center," *Hospital and Community Psychiatry*, 30:540–543.

Galton, L. 1955. "A New Drug Brings Relief for Tense and Anxious," *Cosmopolitan*, August, pp. 82–83.

Gardner, E. 1974, "Implications of Psychoactive Drug Therapy," *New England Journal of Medicine*, 290:800–802.

_____. 1971, "Psychoactive Drug Utilization," *Journal of Drug Issues*, 1:295–300.

Gerard, R. 1957, "Meetings and Societies," *Science*, 125:201–203.

Gewirtz, H., and Graham, S. 1970, "Pharmaceuticals: Valley of the Lies," *Transactions*, 7:5, 8–9.

Gilderman, A. 1979, "Psychopharmacology for Practicing Pharmacists," Hoffmann-LaRoche, Education Brochure, pp. 1–11.

Giordano, F. 1977, "The Benzodiazepines: Pro or Con," *Military Medicine*, 8:629–631.

Glatt, M. 1967, "Benzodiazepines," *British Medical Journal*, 2:1444.

Gold, M., Pottash, M., Extein, I., and Sweeney, D. 1981, "Diagnosis of Depression in the 1980's," *Journal of the American Medical Association*, 245:1562–1564.

Goldberg, D., and Blackwell, B. 1970, "Psychiatric Illness in General Practice. A Detailed Study Using a New Method of Case Identification," *British Medical Journal*, 2:439–443.

Goldberg, D., Cooper, B., Eastwood, M., Kedward, H., and Shepherd, M. 1970, "A Standardized Psychiatric Interview for Use in Community Surveys," *British Journal of the Preventive Society of Medicine*, 24:18–23.

Goldberg, D., Haas, M., Eaton, J., and Grubbs, J. 1976, "Psychiatry and the Primary Care Physician," *Journal of the American Medical Association*, 236:944–945.

Good Housekeeping. 1974, "When Tranquilizers Are Dangerous," October, pp. 187–188.

Good Housekeeping. 1968, "How Can Drugs Affect Mental Health?" January, p. 171.

Good Housekeeping. 1967, "Drugs: A Guide to Using Medications Safely," January, p. 140.

Good Housekeeping. 1963, "The Better Way," October, pp. 159–161.

Gordon, A. 1957. "Happiness Doesn't Come in Pills," *Readers Digest*, January 1, pp. 60–62.

Gottlieb, R. 1978, "The Physician's Knowledge of Psychotropic Drugs: Preliminary Results," *American Journal of Psychiatry*, 15:29–32.

Gottschalk, L., Bates, D., and Fox, R. 1970, "Psychoactive Drug Use," *Archives of General Psychiatry*, 25:395–397.

Gottschalk, L., McGuire, F., Heiser, J., Dinovo, E., and Birch, H. 1979, "A Review of Psychoactive Drug Involved in Deaths in Nine Major United States Cities," *International Journal of the Addictions*, 14:735–758.

Grant, I. 1969, "Drug Habituation in an Urban General Practice," *General Practitioners' Forum*, 202:428–430.

Gray, R., and Smith, M. 1984, "Is Criticism of Tranquilizer Advertising Justified?" *Medical Marketing and Media*, 18:50.

Green, G. 1963. "Too Many Tranquilizers?" *Better Homes and Gardens*, May, p. 46.

Greenblatt, D., and Shader, R. 1976. "Psychopharmacokinetics." In *Clinical Pharmacy and Clinical Pharmacology*, edited by W. Gouveia. New York: North Holland Publishing Co, pp. 3–15.

_____. 1974a. "Introduction." In *Benzodiazepines in Clinical Practice*. New York: Raven Press, pp. 1–10.

_____. 1974b, "Drug Therapy Review," "Rational Use of Psychotropic Drugs," "Anxiety Agents," *American Journal of Hospital Pharmacy*, 31:1077–1080.

_____. 1974c. *Benzodizepines in Clinical Practice*. New York: Raven Press.

_____. 1974d, "Benzodiazepines," *New England Journal of Medicine*, 290:1011–1015.

_____. 1974e, "Benzodiazepines (2nd of 2 parts)," *New England Journal of Medicine*, 291:1239–1243.

_____. 1971, "Meprobamate: A Study of Irrational Drug Use," *American Journal of Psychiatry*, 127:1297–1303.

Greenblatt, D., Woo, Allen, M., Orsulak, P., and Shader, R. 1978, "Rapid Recovery from Massive Diazepam Overdose," *Journal of the American Medical Association*, 240:1872–1874.

Greenblatt, D., Shader, R., and Koch-Wesser, J. 1975, "Psychotropic Drug Use in the Boston Area," *Archives of General Psychiatry*, 32:518–521.

Grob, G.'1977. "The Social History of Medicine and Disease in America: Problems and Possibilities." In *The Medicine Show*, edited by P. Branca. New York: Science History Publications, pp. 63–68.

Halberstam, M. 1980. "T.V.'s Unhealthy Approach to Health News," *T. V. Guide*, December 7, p. 28.

Hammond, K., and Joyce, C. 1975. *Psychoactive Drugs and Social Judgment*. New York: John Wiley and Sons.

Harding, T., and Chrusciel, T. 1975, "The Use of Psychotropic Drugs in Developing Countries," *Bulletin of World Health Organization*, 52:359–367.

Harkins, E. 1978, "Effects of Empty Nest Transition on Self Report of Psychological and Physical Well-Being," *Journal of Marriage and the Family*, 39:549–556.

Harris, T. 1960, "Methaminodiazepoxide," *Journal of the American Medical Association*, 172:1162–1163.

Hartley, W. 1962. "What You Should Know About Tranquilizers," *Reader's Digest*, July, pp. 91–94.

Hasday, J., and Karch, F. 1981, "Benzodiazepine Prescribing in a Family Medicine Center," *Journal of the American Medical Association*, 246:1321–1325.

Hayman, M. 1964, "Science, Mysticism and Psychopharmacology," *California Medicine*, 101:266–271.

Hayman, M., and Ditman, K. 1966, "Influence of Age and Orientation of Psychiatrists on Their Use of Drugs," *Comprehensive Psychiatry*, 7:152–165.

Hecht, A. 1978, "Tranquilizers: Use, Abuse, and Dependency," *FDA Consumer*, 12:21–23.

Helgason, T., and Asmundsson, G. 1980, "Prevalence of Mental Disorders: A 5-Year Follow-Up Study with Questionnaires," *Acta Psychiatrica Scandinavia*, 62:61–67.

Helman, C. 1981, "Tonic, Fuel and Food: Social and Symbolic Aspects of the Long Term Use of Psychotropic Drugs," *Social Science and Medicine*, 15B:521–533.

Hemminki, E. 1982, "Problems in the Measurement of Psychotropic Drug Consumption," *American Journal of Hospital Pharmacy*, 39:325–329.

_____. 1974a, "General Practitioners' Indications for Psychotropic Drugs," *Scandinavian Journal of Social Medicine*, 2:79–85.

_____. 1974b, "Effect of a Doctor's Personal Characteristics and Working Circumstances on the Prescribing of Psychotropic Drugs," *Medical Care*, 12:351–357.

Hemminki, E., and Falkum, E. 1980, "Psychotropic Drug Registration in the

Scandinavian Countries: The Role of Clinical Trials," *Social Science and Medicine*, 14A:547–559.

Hesbacher, P. 1980, "Psychiatric Illness in Family Practice," *Journal of Clinical Psychiatry*, 41:6–10.

Hesbacher, P., and Rickels, K. 1978. "Psychotropic Drug Prescription in General Medical Practice." In *Principles of Psychopharmacology*, edited by W. Clark and J. del Guidice, pp. 615–627. New York: Academic Press.

Hesbacher, P., Rickels, K., Downing, R., and Stepansky, P. 1978, "Assessment of Psychiatric Illness Severity by Family Physicians," *Social Science and Medicine*, 12:45–47.

Hesbacher, P., Rickels, K., and Goldberg, D. 1975a, "Social Factors and Neurotic Symptoms in Family Practice," *American Journal of Public Health*, 65:148–155.

Hesbacher, P., Rickels, K., Gordon, P., Gray, B., Meckelberg, R., Weise, C., and Vandervort, W. 1970, "Setting, Patient, and Doctor Effects on Drug Response in Neurotic Patients," *Psychopharmacologia*, 18:180–208.

Hesbacher, P., Rickels, K., Rial, W., Segal, A., and Zamostein, B. 1976, "Psychotropic Drug Prescription in Family Practice," *Comprehensive Psychiatry*, 17:607–615.

Hesbacher, P., Schein, L., and Leopold, R. 1975b, "Psychiatric Illness Detection: A Comparison of Osteopaths and M.D.'s in Private Family Practice," *Social Science and Medicine*, 9:461–468.

Hill, S. 1977, "Drugs and the Medicalization of Human Problems," *Social Science and Medicine*, 9:461–468.

Himwich, H. 1958, "Psychopharmacologic Drugs," *Science*, 127:59–171.

Hodgins, E. 1956. "The Search Has Only Started." *Life*, October 22, p. 126.

Hoffer, A. 1974, "History of Orthomolecular Psychiatry," *Orthomolecular Psychiatry*, 3:223–230.

Hollister, L. 1980a, "A Look at the Issues," *Psychosomatics*, 21:3–8.

———. 1980b, "Summary," *Psychosomatics*, 21:32.

———. 1976. "Polypharmacy in Psychiatry: Is It Necessary, Good or Bad?" In *Rational Pharmacology and the Right to Treatment*, edited by F. J. Ayd, pp. 19–28. Baltimore: Ayd Medical Communications.

———. 1975, "Drugs for Emotional Disorders," *Journal of the American Medical Association*, 234:942.

———. 1973a, "Anxiety Drugs in Clinical Practice." In *The Benzodiazepines*, edited by S. Garattini, E. Mussini, and L. Randall, pp. 367–377. New York: Raven Press.

———. 1973b, *Clinical Use of Psychotherapeutic Drugs*. Springfield: Charles C Thomas.

Hordern, A. 1962, "The Tranquilizer Problem," *Science Digest*, 52:76–84.

Hornbrook, M. 1977, "Prescription Drugs: Problems for Public Policy," *Current History*, 72:215–224.

Horrobin, D. 1980, "The Valium and Breast Cancer Affair: Lessons Relating to the Involvement of Women in Health Care Research and Policy," *International Journal of Women's Studies*, 4:19–26.

Howie, J. 1979, "The Doctor and the Prescription Pad," *Journal of the Irish Medical Association*, 72:11–14.

Howie, J., and Bigg, A. 1980, "Family Trends in Psychotropic and Antibiotic Prescribing in General Practice," *British Medical Journal*, 22:836–838.

Hubbard, B., and Kripke, D. 1976, "Hypnotic and Minor Tranquilizer Use Among In-Patients and After Discharge," *International Journal of the Addictions*, 11:403–408.

Hubbard, S. 1979, "The Happiness Pushers," *Humanist*, 39:39–42.

Hull, J. 1979, "Psychiatric Referrals in General Practice," *Archives of General Psychiatry*, 36:406–408.

(Humphrey) 1963, "Interagency Coordination in Drug Research and Regulation." Hearings before the (Senate) Subcommittee on Reorganization and International Organizations of the Committee on Government Operations, Washington, D.C., Part 4.

Hussey, H. 1974, "Drugs for Anxiety," *Journal of the American Medical Association*, 228:875.

Ilfeid, F. 1980, "Age, Stressors, and Psychosomatic Disorders," *Psychosomatics*, 21:54–64.

Ingman, S., Lawson, I., Pierpaoli, P., and Blake, P. 1975, "A Survey of the Prescribing and Administration of Drugs in a Long-Term Care Institution for the Elderly," *Journal of the American Geriatrics Society*, 23:309–316.

Irwin, S. 1974, "The Uses and Relative Hazard Potential of Psychoactive Drugs," *Menninger Clinic Bulletin*, 38:15–49.

_____. 1972. *Search for New Drugs*. New York: Marcel Dekker.

Iswarian, V. 1968, "Psychopharmacological Agents: Tranquility or Morbidity Inducers?" *Journal of the Indian Medical Association*, 50:367–371.

Jacobs, D. 1971, "The Psychoactive Drug Thing: Coping or Cop Out?" *Journal of Drug Issues*, 1:264–268.

Jalali, B., Jalali, M., and Turner, F. 1969, "Attitudes Toward Mental Illness," *Journal of Mental and Nervous Disease*, 166:692–700.

(Jarman) 1970, "Drug Abuse Control Amendments—1970." Hearings before the (House) Subcommittee on Public Health and Welfare of the Committee on Interstate and Foreign Commerce, Washington, D.C., Part 2.

Jinks, M. 1977, "Contemporary Drugs in the Management of Anxiety," *Journal of the American Pharmaceutical Association*, NS17:287–290.

Johnstone, E., Owens, D., Frith, C., McPherson, K., Dowie, C., Riley, G., and Gold, A. 1980, "Neurotic Illness and Its Response to Anxiolytic and Antidepressant Treatment," *Psychological Medicine*, 10:321–328.

Kamberg, C. 1982. *Conceptualization and Measurement of Health for Adults*. Santa Monica: Rand Corporation, pp. 1–86.

Kato, G. 1979. "Screening Drugs for Treating Mental Ailments." *Battelle Today: A Battelle Special Report*, pp. 1–4.

Katz, R. 1972, "Drug Therapy—Sedatives and Tranquilizers," *New England Journal of Medicine*, 286:757–760.

Kaufman, A., and Brickner, P. 1973, "Tranquilizer Control," *Journal of the American Medical Association*, 224:1190.

246 / SMALL COMFORT

Kaufman, A., Brickner, P., Varner, R., and Mashburn, W. 1972, "Tranquilizer Control," *Journal of the American Medical Association*, 221:1504–1506.

Keeler, M., and McCurdy, R. 1975, "Medical Practice Without Anti-Anxiety Drugs," *American Journal of Psychiatry*, 132:654–655.

(Kefauver) 1960, "Administered Prices." Hearings before the (Senate) Subcommittee on Antitrust and Monopoly of the Committee on the Judiciary, Washington, D.C., Part 16.

(Kennedy) 1979, "Use and Misuse of Benzodiazepines." Hearings before the (Senate) Subcommittee on Health and Scientific Research on the Committee on Labor and Human Resources, Washington, D.C.

(Kennedy) 1974, "Examination of the Pharmaceutical Industry." Hearings before the (Senate) Subcommittee on Health of the Committee on Labor and Public Welfare, Washington, D.C., Part 2.

Kessler, R., Brown, R., and Bowman, C. 1981, "Sex Differences in Psychiatric Helpseeking: Evidence from Four Large-Scale Surveys," *Journal of Health and Social Behavior*, 22:49–64.

Khavari, K., and Douglass, F. 1980, "Empirically-Derived Hierarchy of Use for Psychotropics: A Cost Benefit Index," *Journal of Drug Education*, 10:325–330.

King, E. 1980, "Sex Bias in Psychoactive Drug Advertisements," *Psychiatry*, 43:129–137.

Klein, D. 1975. "Who Should Not Be Treated with Neuroleptics but Often Are." In *Rational Pharmacology and the Right to Treatment*, edited by F. Ayd, pp. 29–36. Baltimore: Ayd Medical Communications.

Klerman, G. 1975, "Neuroleptics: Too Many or Too Few?" In *Rational Pharmacology and the Right to Treatment*, edited by F. Ayd, pp. 1–18. Baltimore: Ayd Medical Communications.

———. 1971, "A Reaffirmation of the Efficacy of Psychoactive Drugs: A Response to Turner," *Journal of Drug Issues*, 1:312–320.

———. 1970, "Drugs and Social Values," *International Journal of the Addictions*, 5:313–319.

———. 1960, "Sociopsychological Characteristic Use of Drug Therapy," *American Journal of Psychiatry*, 117:111–117.

Klerman, G., and Hirschfeld, R. 1979, "The Use of Antidepressants in Clinical Practice," *Journal of the American Medical Association*, 240:1403–1406.

Kline, N. S. 1976, "Antidepressant Medications," *Journal of the American Medical Association*, 227:1158–1160.

———. 1971. "Manipulation of Life Patterns with Drugs." In *Psychotropic Drugs in the Year 2000*, edited by W. O. Evans and N. S. Kline. Springfield: Charles C Thomas, pp. 69–85.

Koch, H. 1983, "Drug Utilization in Office-Based practice, 1981," Hyattsville: National Center for Health Statistics.

Koch, H. 1982, "Drugs Most Frequently Used in Office-Based Practice: National Ambulatory Medical Care Survey 1980," National Center for Health Statistics, pp. 1–12.

Koch, H., and Campbell, H. 1983, "Utilization of Psychotropic Drugs in Office-

Based Ambulatory Care," National Center for Health Statistics Advance Data, No. 90, U. S. Department of Health and Human Services.

Koran, L. 1979, "Psychiatric Manpower Ratios," *Archives of General Psychiatry*, 36:1409–1415.

Koumjian, K. 1981, "The Use of Valium as a Form of Social Control," *Social Science and Medicine*, 15E:245–249.

Krantz, J., and Carr, C. 1958, *The Pharmacologic Principles of Medical Practice*, (4th ed.). Baltimore: Williams and Wilkins.

Kunnes, R. 1973, "Poly-Drug Abuse: Drug Companies and Doctors," *American Journal of Orthopsychiatry*, 43:530–532.

Ladies Home Journal. 1976, "Women and Tranquilizers," November, pp. 164–167.

Ladimer, I. 1975. "Rational Psychopharmacotherapy and Judicial Interpretations of the Right to Treatment: An Outline." In *Rational Pharmacology and the Right to Treatment*, edited by F. Ayd, pp. 62–90. Baltimore: Ayd Medical Communications.

Langer, E. 1965, "Congress and Drugs: Political Interest in Drug Problems Is Lowest Point in Five Years," *Science*, 147:846–848.

Larned, D. 1975, "Do You Take Valium?" *MS*, 4:26–30.

Lasagna, L., ed. 1980, *Controversies in Therapeutics*. Philadelphia: W. B. Saunders.

Lasagna, L. 1977, "The Role of Benzodiazepines in Nonpsychiatric Medical Practice," *American Journal of Psychiatry*, 134:656–658.

Laties, V., and Weiss, B. 1958, "A Critical Review of the Efficacy of Meprobamate (Miltown, Equanil) in the Treatment of Anxiety," *Journal of Chronic Diseases*, 7:500–519.

Leake, C. 1970. "The Long Road from Drug Abuse to Use." In *Discoveries in Biological Psychiatry*, edited by F. Ayd, pp. 68–84. Philadelphia: J. B. Lippincott.

Lear, J. (ed.). 1960, "Do We Need a Census of Worthless Drugs?" *Saturday Review*, May 7, pp. 53–58.

Learoyd, B. 1974, "Psychotropic Drugs—Are They Justified?" *Medical Journal of Australia*, 1:474–479.

Lech, S., Friedman, G., and Ury, H. 1975, "Characteristics of Heavy Users of Outpatient Prescription Drugs," *Clinical Toxicology*, 8:599–610.

Lehmann, H. 1977, "Drugs of the Future." In *Psychotherapeutic Drugs, Part II*, edited by E. Usdin and I. Forrest, pp. 1469–1489. New York: Marcel Dekker.

Lennard, H., and Bernstein, A. 1974, "Perspectives of the New Psychoactive Drug Technology." In *Social Aspects of the Medical Use of Psychoactive Drugs*. Toronto: ARF Books, pp. 149–155.

Lennard, H., Epstein, L., Bernstein, and Ransom, D. 1971, *Mystification and Drug Misuse*. San Francisco: Jossey-Bass.

Lennard, H., Epstein, L., Bernstein, A., and Ransom, D. 1970, "Hazards Implicit in Prescribing Psychoactive Drugs," *Science*, 169:438–440.

Lennard, H., Epstein, L., and Katzung, B. 1967, "Psychoactive Drug Action and

Group Interaction Process," *Journal of Nervous and Mental Disease*, 145:69–78.

Lesse, S. 1976, "The Preventive Psychiatry of the Future," *Futurist*, 10:228–233.

Lewin, L. 1931, Phantastica, Narcotic and Stimulating Drugs. London: Kegan, Paul.

Lewis, D. 1971, "The Physician's Contribution to the Drug Abuse Scene," *Tufts Medical Alumni Bulletin*, 30:36–39.

Life. 1963, "The Chemical Mind-Changers," March 15, pp. 81–82.

Life. 1954, "Good Medicine from Medicine Man," June 28, p. 101.

Linn, L. 1971, "Physician Characteristics and Attitudes Toward Legitimate Use of Psychotherapeutic Drugs," *Journal of Health and Social Behavior*, 12:132–139.

Linn, L., and Davis, M. 1972, "Physicians' Orientation Toward the Legitimacy of Drug Use and Their Preferred Source of New Drug Information," *Social Science and Medicine*, 6:199–203.

———. 1971, "The Use of Psychotherapeutic Drugs by Middle-Aged Women," *Journal of Health and Social Behavior*, 12:331–340.

Lion, J. et al. 1979, "Psychiatrists' Contribution to the Drug Abuse Scene," *Social Science and Medicine*, 13A:123–125.

Lipowski, L. 1976. "Psychosomatic Medicine: An Overview." In *Modern Trends in Psychosomatic Medicine*, edited by O. Hill, pp. 1–20. Boston: Butterworths.

Locke, B., and Garner, E. 1969, "Psychiatric Disorders Among the Patients of General Practitioners and Internists" *Public Health Reports*, 84:167–173.

Logerfo, J. 1974, "The Impact of a Formulary Change Restricting Minor Tranquilizers: The Washington State Medicaid Experience." Unpublished paper.

Loomis, T., and West, T. 1957, "Comparative Sedative Effects of a Barbiturate and Some Tranquilizer Drugs on Normal Subjects," *Sedation in Normal Subjects*, 122:525–531.

Mackowiak, J. 1983, "The Effect of Advertising and Promotion on Primary and Selective Demand in the Pharmaceutical Industry." Ph.D. dissertation, University of North Carolina.

Madsen, B., Murphy, B., and Wearne, K. 1979, "Drug Usage in a Western Rural Community," *Australian and New Zealand Journal of Medicine*, 9:269–274.

Mahoney, T. 1959. *The Merchants of Life*. New York: Harper and Brothers.

Maletzky, B., and Klotter, J. 1976, "Addiction to Diazepam," *International Journal of the Addictions*, 11:95–115.

Mandersheid, R. 1976, "Mental Health and the Future," *Futures*, 8:331–335.

Manheimer, D., Davidson, S., Balter, M., Mellinger, G., Cisin, I., and Parry, H. 1973, "Popular Attitudes and Beliefs About Tranquilizers," *American Journal of Psychiatry*, 130:1246.

Manheimer, D., Mellinger, G., and Balter, M. 1968, "Psychotherapeutic Drugs," *California Medicine*, 109:445–451.

Mant, A., and Darroch, D. 1975, "Media Images and Medical Images," *Social Science and Medicine*, 9:613–618.

Marcus, A., and Seeman, T. 1981, "Sex Differences in Reports of Illness and Disability: A Preliminary Test of the Fixed Role Obligations 'Hypothesis'," *Journal of Health and Social Behavior*, 22:174–182.

Marks, J. 1981, "The Benzodiazepines—Use and Abuse: Current Status," *Pharmacy International*, 2:84–87.

_____. 1972, *The Benzodiazepines*. Baltimore: University Press.

Maronde, R., Burks, D., Lee, P., Licht, P., McCarron, M., McCary, M., and Serbert, S. 1969, "Physician Prescribing Practices," *American Journal of Hospital Pharmacy*, 26:566–573.

Maronde, R., Lee, P., McCarron, M., and Seibert, S. 1971, "A Study of Prescribing Patterns," *Medical Care*, 9:383–395.

Martin, R., Roberts, W., and Clayton, P. 1980, "Psychiatric Status After Hysterectomy," *Journal of the American Medical Association*, 244:350–354.

Mathew, R., Largen, J., and Claghorn, J. 1979, "Biological Symptoms of Depression," *Psychosomatic Medicine*, 41:439–443.

Mawson, A., and Jacobs, K. 1978, "Corn Consumption, Tryptophan, and Cross-National Homicide Rates," *Journal of Orthomolecular Psychiatry*, 7:227–230.

May, C. 1961, "Selling Drugs by Educating Physicians," *Journal of Medical Education*, 63:1–23.

Mayfield, D., and Morrison, D. 1973, "The Use of Minor Tranquilizers in a Teaching Hospital," *Southern Medical Journal*, 66:589–592.

McCalls. 1976, "Tranquilizers: Their Use and Abuse," May, pp. 94–95.

McClean, L. 1976, "What's Good About Tranquilizers." *Vogue*, April, p. 221.

McCranie, E., Horowitz, A., and Marin, R. 1978, "Alleged Sex-Role Stereotyping in the Assessment of Women's Physical Complaints: A Study of General Practitioners," *Social Science and Medicine*, 12:111–116.

McGee, A. 1979. "Your Neighborhood Dr. Feelgood." *Commercial Appeal*, October 14, p. G1.

McGuire, F., Birch, H., Gottschalk, L., Heiser, J., and Dinovo, E. 1976, "A Comparison of Suicide and Non-Suicide Deaths Involving Psychotropic Drugs in Four Major U. S. Cities," *American Journal of Public Health*, 66:1058–1061.

McNair, D. 1973, "Anti-Anxiety Drugs and Human Performance," *Archives of General Psychiatry*, 29:611–617.

McRee, C., Corder, B., and Haizlip, T. 1974, "Psychiatrists' Responses to Sexual Bias in Pharmaceutical Advertising," *American Journal of Psychiatry*, 131:1273–1275.

Mechanic, D. 1978a, "Explanations of Mental Illness," *Journal of Nervous and Mental Disorders*, 166:381–386.

_____. 1978b, "Sex, Illness, Illness Behavior and the Use of Health Services," *Social Science and Medicine*, 12B:207–214.

250 / SMALL COMFORT

Meerloo, J. 1955, "Medication into Submission—The Danger of Therapeutic Coercion," *Journal of Nervous and Mental Disease*, 122:353–360.

Mellinger, G. 1974. "The Psychotherapeutic Drug Scene in San Francisco." In *Drug Abuse: Data and Debate*, edited by P. Blachly, pp. 226–240. Springfield: Charles C Thomas.

———, 1971, "Psychotherapeutic Drug Use Among Adults: A Model for Young Drug Users," *Journal of Drug Issues*, 1:274–293.

Mellinger, G. D., Balter, M. B., Manheimer, D. I., Cisin, I. H., and Parry, H. J. 1978, "Psychic Distress, Life Crisis and Use of Psychotherapeutic Medications," *Archives of General Psychiatry*, 35:1045–1051.

Mellinger, G., Balter, M., and Manheimer, D. 1971, "Patterns of Psychotherapeutic Drug Use Among Adults in San Francisco," *Archives of General Psychiatry*, 25:385–394.

Mellinger, G., Balter, M., Parry, H., Manheimer, D., and Cisin, I. 1974. "An Overview of Psychotherapeutic Drug Use in the United States." In *Drug Use: Epidemiological and Sociological Approaches*, edited by E. Josephson and E. Carroll, pp. 333–336. Washington, D.C.: Hemisphere Publishers.

Melville, A., and Johnson, C. 1982. *Cured to Death*. London: Secker and Warburg.

Meyer, R. 1957, "Tranquilizer and Traffic," *Science Digest*, 42:69–73.

Miller, M. 1979, "Mental Illness and the Problems of Boundaries." In *Medicine in the Public Interest*, edited by M. Schworm, pp. 1–24. Washington, D.C.

Miller, R. 1974, "Prescribing Habits of Physicians," *Drug Intelligence and Clinical Pharmacy*, 8:81.

Milliren, J. 1977, "Some Contingencies Affecting the Utilization of Tranquilizers in Long Term Care of the Elderly," *Journal of Health and Social Behavior*, 18:206–211.

Mintz, M. 1965. *The Therapeutic Nightmare*. Boston: Houghton Mifflin.

Morgan, A. 1973, "Minor Tranquilizers, Hypnotics and Sedatives," *American Journal of Nursing*, 73:1220–1222.

Morgan, J. 1980. "The Politics of Medication." In *Controversies in Therapeutics*, edited by L. Lasagna. Philadelphia: W. B. Saunders, pp. 16–22.

Morris, L., and Kanouse, D. 1981, "Consumer Reactions to the Tone of Written Drug Information," *American Journal of Hospital Pharmacy*, 38:667–669.

Mosher, E. 1976, "Portrayal of Women in Drug Advertising: A Medical Betrayal," *Journal of Drug Issues*, 6:72–78.

Moskowitz, M. 1960, "Librium: A Marketing Case History," *Drug and Cosmetic Industry*, 87:460–461, 566–567.

MS. 1975, "The Selling of Valium," November, pp. 34–35.

Muller, C. 1972, "The Overmedicated Society: Forces in the Marketplace for Medical Care," *Science*, 176:488.

Mundy, G., Fleckenstein, L., Mazzullo, J., Sundaresan, P., Weintraub, M., and Lasagna, L. 1974, "Current Medical Practice and the Food and Drug Administration," *Journal of the American Medical Association*, 229:1744–1748.

Munro, A. 1969, "Psychiatric Illness in Gynecological Outpatients: A Preliminary Study," *British Journal of Psychiatry*, 115:807–809.

Myers, J., and Weissman, M. 1980, "Psychiatric Disorders and Their Treatment," *Medical Care*, 18:117–123.

Najman, J., Klein, D., and Munro, C. 1982, "Patient Characteristics Negatively Stereotyped by Doctors," *Social Science and Medicine*, 16:1781–1789.

Nathanson, C. 1980, "Social Roles and Health Status Among Women: The Significance of Employment," *Social Science and Medicine*, 14A:463–471.

———. 1975, "Illness and the Feminine Role: A Theoretical Review," *Social Science and Medicine*, 9:57.

(Nelson) 1976, "Competitive Problems in the Drug Industry." Hearings before the (Senate) Subcommittee on Monopoly of the Select Committee on Small Business, Washington, D.C., Part 30.

(Nelson) 1971, "Advertising of Proprietary Medicines." Hearings before the (Senate) Subcommittee on Monopoly of the Select Committee on Small Business, Washington, D.C., Part 2.

(Nelson) 1969, "Competitive Problems in the Drug Industry." Hearings before the (Senate) Subcommittee on Monopoly of the Select Committee on Small Business, Washington, D.C., Part 13.

Newmark, C. 1971, "Techniques Used to Assess the Efficacy of Psychotropic Drugs: A Critical Review," *Psychological Reports*, 28:715–723.

New Republic. 1957, "Domestic Tranquility," June 24, pp. 5–6.

Newsweek. 1979, "Drugs and Psychiatry," November 12, pp. 98–104.

Newsweek. 1964a, "Dornwal in the Dock," September 7, p. 59.

Newsweek. 1964b, "Tranquility and After," April 20, p. 110.

Newsweek. 1960, "Investigation: Pills," February 1, p. 66.

Newsweek. 1958, "Pills and a Probe," March 10, p. 65.

Newsweek. 1957, "Pills and Perils," May 6, p. 105.

Newsweek. 1956b, "Putting Tranquilizers to the Test," September 29, p. 36.

Newsweek. 1956a, "'Ideal' in Tranquility," October 29, pp. 63–64.

Newsweek. 1956c, "Pills vs. Worry/How Goes the Frantic Quest," May 21, pp. 68–70.

Newsweek. 1956d, "Sobering Up," January 1, p. 64.

New Yorker. 1968, "Annals of Medicine: The Case of Mrs. Carter," December 7, pp. 207–208.

Nielsen, A., and Williams, T. 1980, "Depression in Ambulatory Medical Patients," *Archives of General Psychiatry*, 37:999–1004.

Nielsen, J. A., Henriksen, T., and Nielsen, J. 1980, "Psychiatric Illness and Use of Psychotropic Drugs in Geographically Delimited Population of Samso, Denmark," *Acta Psychiatrica Scandinavia*, 62:97–102.

Nightingale, S., Dormer, R., and Dupont, R. 1975, "Inappropriate Prescribing of Psychoactive Drugs," *Annals of Internal Medicine*, 83:896–898.

Nimb, M. 1980, "Psychiatry and Primary Health Services in Developing and Developed Countries," *Acta Psychiatrica Scandinavia*, 62:103–111.

Norman, M. 1974, "Calm Down-At-Your Own Risk," *Today's Health*, 52:16–19.

Nowes, R. 1980, "The Prognosis of Anxiety Neurosis," *Archives of General Psychiatry*, 37:173–178.

Olafsson, O., Sigfusson, S., and Grimsson, A. 1980, "Control of Addictive Drugs in

Iceland 1976–78," *Journal of Epidemiology and Community Health*, 34:305–308.

Osmond, H., Mullaly, R., and Bisbee, C. 1978, "The Medical Model and the Responsible Patient," *Hospital and Community Psychiatry*, 29:522–524.

Overall, J., Henry, B., Markett, J., and Emken, R. 1972, "Decisions About Drug Therapy," *Archives of General Psychiatry*, 26:140–145.

Palumbo, F., and Framm, H. "A Study of the Extent of Anti-Anxiety Drug Use in Nursing Homes." Presented at the American Pharmaceutical Association Annual Meeting, April 1979.

Parish, P. 1974, "Sociology of Prescribing," *British Medical Journal*, 30:214–217.

———. 1973, "What Influences Have Led to Increased Prescribing of Psychotropic Drugs?" *Journal of the Royal College of General Practitioners*, 23:49–57.

Parry, H. 1971, "Patterns of Psychotropic Drug Use Among American Adults," *Journal of Drug Issues*, 1:269–273.

———. 1968, "Use of Psychotropic Drugs by U. S. Adults," *Public Health Reports*, 83:799–810.

Parry, H., Balter, M., and Cisin, I. 1970–71, "Primary Levels of Underreporting Psychosomatic Drug Use," *Public Opinion Quarterly*, 34:582–592.

Parry, H., Balter, M., Mellinger, G., Cisin, I., and Manheimer, D. 1973, "National Patterns of Psychotherapeutic Drug Use," *Archives of General Psychiatry*, 28:769–783.

Parry, H., Cisin, I., Balter, M., Mellinger, G., and Manheimer, D. et al. n.d., "Increasing Alcohol Intake as a Coping Mechanism for Psychic Distress." Paper-Social Research Group, George Washington University.

Parry, H., Manheimer, D., and Balter, M. 1978, "Psychotherapeutic Agents: Patient Attitudes and National Patterns of Use." National Institute of Mental Health, May 1978.

Pearlin, L. 1962, "Treatment Values and Enthusiasm for Drugs in a Mental Hospital," *Psychiatry*, 25:170–179.

Peet, M., and Moonie, L. 1979, "Abuse of Benzodiazepines," *British Medical Journal*, 1:714.

Pekkanen, J. 1975, "The Tranquilizer Way," *New Republic*, 173:17.

Pevnick, J., Jasinski, D., and Haertzen, C. 1978, "Abrupt Withdrawal from Therapeutically Administered Diazepam," *Archives of General Psychiatry*, 35:995–998.

Pflanz, M., Basler, H., and Schwoon, D. 1977, "Use of Tranquilizing Drugs by a Middle-aged Population in a West German City," *Journal of Health and Social Behavior*, 18:194–205.

PMA Newsletter. 1982a, "HGR Defends Generic Use of Brand Name Valium," May 10, p. 5.

PMA Newsletter. 1982b, "Roche Sues Nader Group for Misuse of Valium Trademark," May 3, p. 5.

PMA Newsletter. 1981, "First Annual Summary of Drug Use," October 26, pp. 1–3.

BIBLIOGRAPHY / 253

Popkin, M., MacKenzie, T., and Hall, R. 1980, "Consultee's Concordance with Consultants' Psychotropic Drug Recommendations," *Archives of General Psychiatry*, 37:1017–1021.
Potter, W., and Sargent, M. 1979, "What You Should Know About Psychotropic Drug Treatment," *Pharmacy Times*, 45:29–37.
Prather, J., and Fidell, L. 1975, "Sex Differences in the Content and Style of Medical Advertisements," *Social Science and Medicine*, 3:23–26.
Preskorn, S., and Denner, L. 1977, "Benzodiazepines and Withdrawal Psychosis," *Journal of the American Medical Association*, 237:36–38.
Prient, R., Balter, M., and Caffey, E. 1978, "Hospital Surveys of Prescribing with Psychotherapeutic Drugs," *Archives of General Psychiatry*, 35:1271–1275.
Prince, E. 1978, "Welfare Status, Illness and Subjective Health Definition," *American Journal of Public Health*, 68:865–871.
Rabkin, R. 1980. *Inner and Outer Space*. New York: Norton Publishers.
Radelet, M. 1981, "Health Beliefs, Social Networks, and Tranquilizer Use," *Journal of Health and Social Behavior*, 22:165–173.
Radloff, L. n.d., "Depression and the Empty Nest." Center for Epidemiologic Studies, National Institutes of Mental Health (unpublished).
Radloff, L., and Rae, D. 1979, "Susceptibility and Precipitating Factors in Depression: Sex Differences and Similarities," *Journal of Abnormal Psychology*, 88:174–181.
Raft, D., Davidson, J., Toomey, T., Spencer, R., and Lewis, B. 1975, "Inpatient and Outpatient Patterns of Psychotropic Drug Prescribing by Non-Psychiatrist Physicians," *American Journal of Psychiatry*, 132:1309–1313.
Raley, J. 1957, "That Wonderful Frustrated Feeling," *American Mercury*, July, pp. 20–24.
Randell, L. 1961, "Pharmacology of Chlordiazepoxide (Librium)," *Diseases of the Nervous System*, 22:7–15.
Randell, L., Heise, G., Shallek, W., Bagdon, E., Banziger, R., Boris, R., Mop, R., and Abrams, W. 1961, "Pharmacological and Clinical Studies on Valium: A New Psychotherapeutic Agent of the Benzodiazepine Class," *Current Therapeutic Research*, 3:405–425.
Randell, L., Schallek, W., Heise, G., Keith, E., and Bagdon, R. 1960, "The Psychosedative Properties of Methaminodiazepoxide," *Journal of Pharmacology and Experimental Therapeutics*, 129:163–171.
Rank, S., and Jacobson, C. 1977, "Hospital Nurses' Compliance with Medication Overdose Orders: A Failure to Replicate," *Journal of Health and Social Behavior*, 18:188–193.
Rather, L. 1959, "Courage, Mr. Huxley! ... ", *Nation*, 188:188–189.
Ray, O. 1978. *Drugs, Society and Human Behavior*. St. Louis: C. V. Mosby.
Raynes, N. 1979, "Factors Affecting the Prescribing of Psychotropic Drugs in General Practice Consultations," *Psychological Medicine*, 9:671–679.
_____. 1978, "General Practice Consultation Study: Some Preliminary Observations," *Social Science and Medicine*, 12:311–315.
Renaud, M., Beauchemin, J., Lalonde, L., Poirier, H., and Berthiaume, S. 1980,

"Practice Settings and Prescribing Profiles: The Simulation of Tension Headaches to General Practitioners Working in Different Practice," *American Journal of Public Health*, 70:1068–1073.

Rickels, K. 1980, Proceedings of a Conference. Research Analysis and Utilization System, National Institute on Drug Abuse, Washington, D.C., September.

_____. 1978, "Use of Antianxiety Agents in Anxious Outpatients," *Psychopharmacologia*, 58:1–17.

_____. 1973, "Predictors of Response to Benzodiazepines in Clinical Practice." In *The Benzodiazepines*, edited by S. Garattini, E. Mussini, and L. Randall. New York: Raven Press, pp. 391–404.

_____. 1972, "Drug, Doctor Warmth, and Clinic Setting in the Symptomatic Response to Minor Tranquilizer," *Psychopharmacologia*, 20:20.

Rickels, K., Csanalosi, I., Chung, H., Case, G., and Downing, R. 1974, "Amitriptyline in Anxious-Depression Outpatients: A Controlled Study," *American Journal of Psychiatry*, 131:25–30.

Rickels, K., Garcia, C., Lipman, R., Derogatis, L., and Fisher, E. 1976, "The Hopkins Symptom Checklist—Assessing Emotional Distress in Obstetric-Gynecologic Practice," *Primary Care*, 3:751–764.

Rickels, K., and Hesbacher, P. 1977, "Psychopharmacologic Agents: Prescription Patterns of Non-Psychiatrists," *Psychosomatics*, 17:338–344.

Rickels, K., and Howard, K. 1970, "The Physician Questionnaire: A Useful Tool in Psychiatric Drug Research," *Psychopharmacologia*, 17:338–344.

Riessman, C. 1979, "Interviewer Effects in Psychiatric Epidemiology—A Study of Medical and Lay Interviewers and Their Impact on Reported Symptoms," *American Journal of Public Health*, 69:485–491.

Robinson, J. 1957, "A Chance for the Mentally Ill," *Science News Letter*, 71:266–267.

Robinson, L. 1959, "Happy Pills for Animals," *Coronet*, 46:165–166.

Rogers, J. 1971, "Drug Abuse—Just What the Doctor Ordered," *Psychology Today*, 12:16–24.

Rosenbaum, J. 1982, "Current Concepts in Psychiatry," *Medical Intelligence*, 306:401–404.

Rosenbaum, P. 1977, "The Legal Abuse of Prescription Drugs: Evidence of a Continuing Drug Problem," *Journal of Drug Issues*, 7:123–127.

Rosenberg, S., Berenson, L., Kavaler, F., Govelik, E., and Levine, B. 1974, "Prescribing Patterns in the New York Medicaid Program," *Medical Care*, 7:138–151.

Rosenfeld, A. 1979, "How Anxious Should Science Make Us?" *Saturday Review*, 24:16–21.

Rowe, I. 1973, "Prescriptions by Psychotropic Drugs by General Practitioners: 2. Antidepressant," *Medical Journal of Australia*, 1:642–644.

Rucker, T. "Production and Prescribing of Minor Tranquilizers: A Macro-View." Paper presented to the American Orthopsychiatric Association, April 19, 1980.

Saltzberger, G. 1978, "Office Management of Anxiety," *Behavioral Medicine*, 6:20–23.

Scheff, T. 1976, "Medical Dominance," *American Behavioral Scientist*, 19:309.

Schiff, A., Murphy, J., and Anderson, J. 1975, "Non-Pharmacological Factors in Drug Therapy—The Interactions of Doctor, Patient, and Tablet Appearance in the Treatment of Anxiety/Depressive Syndromes," *Journal of International Medicine Research*, 3:125–133.

Schmidt, A. 1978, "Comment," *American Journal of Psychiatry*, 135:1057–1058.

Science. 1956, "Peace Pills," July 27, p. 167.

Science Digest. 1964a, "Beware Tranquilizer Addiction," March, pp. 40–41.

Science Digest. 1964b, "Your Guide to Mind Drugs," January, p. 69.

Science Digest. 1959, "Tranquilizers Can Hurt Emotional Health," June, p. 37.

Science Digest. 1957, "You Can Be Too Tranquil," August, p. 46.

Science Digest. 1956, "Questions Driving Safety While on Tranquilizers," May, p. 37.

Science Digest. 1955a, "'Drugged' Artists Paint Better," September, p. 35.

Science Digest. 1955b, "How Good Drugs for Mental Illness," July, p. 30.

Science News. 1975, "Tightening the Lid on Legal Drugs," June 14, p. 382.

Science News. 1973, "Catch 22 of Psychopharmacology," September 22, pp. 389–390.

Science News. 1967a, "More on Drug Abuse," March 11, p. 232.

Science News. 1967b, "FDA Gets Miltown Ruling," February, p. 185.

Science News. 1966a, "Miltown's Effect on Brain a Mystery," July 9, p. 24.

Science News. 1966b, "Mind Drugs Puzzling," May 17, p. 196.

Science News Letter. 1963, "Thirty Leading Drugs Buried in Medical Time Capsule," October 12, p. 231.

Science News Letter. 1960a, "Prescribing Tranquilizers Called Doctors' Disease," February 6, p. 89.

Science News Letter. 1960b, "Tranquilizers Cost Us $280,000,000 Each Year," January 30, p. 73.

Science News Letter. 1959a, "Tranquilizer May Not Be Habit Forming," March 8, p. 153.

Science News Letter. 1959b, "Tranquilizers Pacify Patient and Doctor," February 28, p. 136.

Science News Letter. 1959c, "Tranquilizers Substituted for Hospitals in Haiti," January 5, p. 5.

Science News Letter. 1958a, "Drug Fights Mental Ills," November 1, p. 275.

Science News Letter. 1958b, "Place of Tranquilizers Still to Be Determined," May 31, p. 347.

Science News Letter. 1957a, "Drug Lowers Blood Pressure and Anxiety," December 15, p. 376.

Science News Letter. 1957b, "Drugs Slow Reactions," May 25, p. 325.

Science News Letter. 1957c, "Tranquilizers Make Pets Easier to Handle," January 19, p. 41.

Science News Letter. 1956a, "Tranquilizer Checks Pregnancy Nausea," December 15, p. 380.

Science News Letter. 1965b, "You Can Drive Tranquilized," November 3, p. 287.

Science News Letter. 1956c, "Relaxing Drugs Will Cause Great Change," October 27, p. 283.

Science News Letter. 1956d, "Mental Cure Rate Increased One-Third," June 23, p. 396.
Science News Letter. 1956e, "Patients Drug Will Help," May 12, p. 303.
Science News Letter. 1956f, "New Drug Is Calming," January 7, p. 7.
Science News Letter. 1954a, "Drug Quiets Mentally Ill," April 3, p. 213.
Science News Letter. 1954b, "Blood Pressure Drug Calms Mental Patients," February 27, p. 130.
Scott, R. 1957, "Don't Misuse Tranquilizers," *Today's Health*, 35:23, 61.
Seidenberg, R. 1974, "Images of Health, Illness and Women in Drug Advertising," *Journal of Drug Issues*, 4:264–267.
———. 1971, "Drug Advertising and Perception of Mental Illness," *Mental Hygiene*, 55:21–31.
Selling, L. 1955, "Clinical Study of a New Tranquilizing Drug," *Journal of the American Medical Association*, 157:1594.
Shader, R., and Greenblatt, D. 1977, "Clinical Implications of Benzodiazepine Pharmacokinetics," *American Journal of Psychiatry*, 134:652–657.
Shader, R., Greenblatt, D., Salzman, C., Kochansky, G., and Harmatz, J. 1975, "Benzodiazepines: Safety and Toxicity," *Psychopharmacology Research Laboratory*, 36:23–26.
Shapiro, S., and Baron, S. 1961, "Prescriptions for Psychotropic Drugs in a Noninstitutional Population," *Public Health Reports*, 76:481–488.
Shepherd, M. 1972, "The Classification of Psychotropic Drugs," *Psychological Medicine*, 2:96–110.
Sheppard, C., Collins, L., Fiorentino, D., Fracchia, J., and Merlis, S. 1969, "Polypharmacy in Psychiatric Treatment: 1. Incidence at a State Hospital," *Current Therapeutic Research*, 11:765–774.
Sheppard, C., Moan, E., Fracchia, J., and Merlis, S. 1975, "Psychiatrists Prescription Practices," *New York State Journal of Medicine*, 75:1327–1333.
Siegal, L. (ed.). 1980, "The Meaning of Medication," *Art of Medication*, 1:1–31.
Silverman, M., Lee, P., and Lydecker, M. 1981, *Pills and the Public Purse.* Los Angeles: University of California Press.
Simmons, H. 1974, "The Role of the Food and Drug Administration in Regulating Drug Advertising," *Journal of Drug Issues*, 4:291–293.
Skegg, D., Doll, R., and Perry, J. 1977, "Use of Medicines in General Practice," *British Medical Journal*, 1:1561–1563.
Skegg, D., Richards, S., and Doll, R. 1979, "Minor Tranquilizers and Road Accidents," *British Medical Journal*, 1:917–919.
Smith, G. 1980, "Viewpoints," Hoffmann-LaRoche Publication, February, pp. 1–5.
Smith, M. 1983, "Lay Periodical Courage of the Minor Tranquilizers: The First Quarter Century," *Pharmacy in History*, 25:131–136.
Smith, M. 1977, "Drug Product Advertising and Prescribing: A Review of the Evidence," *American Journal of Hospital Pharmacy*, 34:1208–1224.
Smith, M., and Griffin, L. 1977, "Rationality of Appeals Used in the Promotion of Psychotropic Drugs: A Comparison of Male and Female Models," *Social Science and Medicine*, 11:409.

Smith, M., and Ryan, M. 1968, "Dissonance and the Physician," *Medical Marketing and Media*, 3:17–19.

Smith, M., Strecker, P., and Hair, J. 1977, "Sex Appeals in Prescription Drug Advertising," *Medical Marketing and Media*, 12:64–72.

Snider, A. 1978. "Tranquilizer Defended." *Commercial Appeal*, October 1, p. C4.

_____. 1969. "The 15 Most Important Drugs." *Science Digest*, September, pp. 72–76.

Solomon, F., White, C. Parron, D., and Mendelson, W. 1979, "Sleeping Pills, Insomnia and Medical Practice," *New England Journal of Medicine*, 300:803–808.

Solow, C. 1975, "Psychotropic Drugs in Somatic Disorders," *International Journal of Psychiatry in Medicine*, 6:267–282.

Sorenson, A., Morgan, J., and Trabert, N. 1978, "The Prescribing of Valium as Health Care Provider Behavior." Paper presented to Medical Sociology Group of the British Sociological Association.

Steen, J. 1963, "The Truth About Brain Drugs." *Popular Science Monthly*, February, pp. 70–73.

Sternbach, L. 1979, "The Benzodiazepine Story," *Journal of Medicinal Chemistry*, 22:1–7.

_____. 1972, "The Discovery of Librium," *Agents and Actions*, 2:193–196.

Stevenson, I. 1957, "Tranquilizers and the Mind," *Harper's*, 215:21–27.

Stewart, T., Joyce, C., and Lindell, M. 1975. "New Analyses: Application of Judgement Theory to Physicians' Judgements of Drug Effects." In *Psychoactive Drugs and Social Judgement*, edited by K. Hammond and C. Joyce. New York: John Wiley and Sons, pp. 110–114.

Stimson, G. 1975a, "Women in a Doctored World," *New Society*, 6:265–267.

_____. 1975b, "The Message of Psychotropic Drug Ads," *Journal of Communication*, 25:153–160.

Stolley, P. 1971, "Cultural Lag in Health Care," *Inquiry*, 8:71–76.

Stolley, P., Becker, M., McEvilla, J., Lasagna, L., Gainor, M., and Sloane, L. 1972, "Drug Prescribing and Use in an American Community," *Annals of Internal Medicine*, 76:537–540.

Stolley, P., and Lasagna, L. 1969, "Prescribing Patterns of Physicians," *Journal of Chronic Diseases*, 22:395–405.

Swenson, W. 1981, "Psychological Correlates of Medical Illness," *Psychosomatics*, 22:384–391.

Snyder, S. 1975, "A Demonology of Dope," *Psychology Today*, 8:88–89.

Taylor, M., Spero, M., Simeon, J., and Fink, M. 1969, "High Dose Chlordiazepoxide Therapy of Anxiety," *Current Therapeutic Research*, 11:9–13.

Temin, P. 1980. *Taking Your Medicine*. Cambridge: Harvard University Press.

Tessler, R., and Mechanic, D. 1978, "Psychological Distress and Perceived Health Status," *Journal of Health and Social Behavior*, 19:254–262.

Tessler, R., Mechanic, D., and Dimond, M. 1976, "The Effect of Psychological

Tessler, R., Stokes, R., and Pietras, M. 1978, "Consumer Response to Valium," *Drug Therapy*, 8:178–183.

Distress on Physician Utilization: A Prospective Study," *Journal of Health and Social Behavior*, 17:353–364.

Thompson, A. 1973, "Prescribing of Hypnotics and Sedatives in New Zealand," *Pharmaceutical Journal of New Zealand*, 35:15.

Time. 1981, "The Skies Grow Friendlier," August 17, p. 43.

Time. 1980a, "Minor Tranquilizers," July 28, p. 33.

Time. 1980b, "Yellow Light for Tranquilizers," July 21, p. 53.

Time. 1980c, "Psychoprofits," January 7, p. 90.

Time. 1979a, "Tranquil Tales," September 24, p. 78.

Time. 1979b, "Puzzling Pills," July 30, p. 70.

Time. 1977, "Miltown? No Martini," June 3, p. 63.

Time. 1965, "Letdown for Miltown," April 30, p. 85.

Time. 1964, "What Tranquilizers Have Done," April 24, pp. 43–44.

Time. 1960a, "Report on Librium," May 30, p. 37.

Time. 1960b, "Too Many Drugs?" April 25, pp. 78, 80.

Time. 1960c, "Tranquil but Alert," March 7, p. 47.

Time. 1960d, "Trouble in Miltown," February 8, p. 83.

Time. 1958a, "Upjohn's Medicine Man," September 15, pp. 65–66.

Time. 1958b, "Drugged Future," February 24, pp. 35–36.

Time. 1958c, "Honorable Tranki," February 17, p. 44.

Time. 1957a, "Miltown? No Martinis!" June 3, p. 48.

Time. 1957b, "Happiness by Prescription," March 11, p. 59.

Time. 1956a, "Pills for the Mind," June 11, p. 54.

Time. 1956b, "Don't-Give-A-Damn-Pills," February 27, p. 98.

Time. 1955, "Pills for the Mind," March 7, pp. 63–64.

Time. 1954, "Wonder Drug of 1954?" June 14, p. 79.

Today's Health. 1960, "The Story of Tranquilizers," November, pp. 32–33.

Transaction. 1969, "Have a Tranquilizer, Dear," May 19, p. 10.

Trethowan, W. 1975, "Pills for Personal Problems," *British Medical Journal*, 3:749–750.

Trute, B., and Loewen, A. 1978, "Public Attitude Toward the Mentally Ill as a Function of Prior Personal Experience," *Social Psychiatry*, 13:79–84.

Tucker, J. 1980. "Psychotropic Drugs: The Mood Makers." *Cosmopolitan*, June, pp. 248, 260–262.

Turner, J. 1971, "A Critical Assessment of Drug Marketing Practices," *Journal of Drug Issues*, 1:301–311.

Tyrer, P. 1974, "The Benzodiazepine Bonanza," *Lancet*, 2:709–710.

Uhlenhuth, E., Balter, M., and Lipman, R. 1978, "Minor Tranquilizers—Clinical Correlates of Use in an Urban Population," *Archives of General Psychiatry*, 35:650–655.

Uhlenhuth, E., Lipman, R., Balter, M., and Stern, M. 1974, "Symptom Intensity and Life Stress in the City," *Archives of General Psychiatry*, 31:759–764.

Vaillant, G., Brighton, J., and McArthur, C. 1970, "Physicians' Use of Mood-Altering Drugs," *New England Journal of Medicine*, 282:365–370.

Vinar, O. 1978, "Psychotropic Drugs: Their Risk-Benefit Ratio," *Aggresologie*, 19:99–102.

Vogue. 1975, "Danger Ahead! Valium—The Pill You Love Can Turn on You," February, 152–153.

Waldron, I. 1977, "Increased Prescribing of Valium, Librium and Other Drugs— An Example of the Influence of Economic and Social Factors on the Practice of Medicine," *International Journal of Health Services,* 1:37–62.

Weatherall, M. 1962, "Tranquilizers," *British Medical Journal,* 1:5287.

Webb, S., and Collette, J. 1975, "Urban Ecological and Household Correlates of Stress-Alleviative Drug Use," *American Behavioral Scientist,* 18:750–770.

Weibert, R., and Dee, D. 1978, "Improving Compliance—Benzodiazepines," *Current Prescribing,* 3:48–50.

Weiner, J., and Schumacher, G. 1976, "Psychotropic Drug Therapy Knowledge of Health Care Practitioners," *American Journal of Hospital Pharmacy,* 33:237–241.

Weiss, B. 1963, "Drugs and Behavior." *Science,* June 7, p. 1109.

Welles, M. 1956, "Your Doctor and You," *Farm Journal,* October, p. 1.

Wheatly, D., and Dalton, K. 1972, "Evaluation of Psychotropic Drugs in General Practice," *Proceedings of the Royal Society of Medicine,* 65:11–14.

Wiersum, J. 1974, "Psychotropic Drugs in Addiction," *Journal of the American Medical Society,* 227:79.

Wilcox, J. 1977, "Psychotherapeutic Prescribing Patterns in General Practice," *New Zealand Medical Journal,* 85:363–366.

Williams, P. 1978, "Physical Ill-Health and Psychotropic Drug Prescription—A Review," *Psychological Medicine,* 8:683–693.

Winkelman, N. 1975. "The Use of Neuroleptic Drugs in the Treatment of Nonpsychotic Psychiatric Patients." In *Rational Pharmacology and the Right to Treatment,* edited by F. Ayd. Baltimore: Ayd Medical Communications, pp. 161–163.

Winstead, D., Lawson, T., and Abbott, D. 1976, "Diazepam Use in Military Sick Call," *Military Medicine,* 141:180.

Wolfe, S. 1981, Letter to Arthur Hull Hayes, June 18.

_____. 1974, "Testimony." Senate Health Subcommittee, February 25.

(Wolff) 1979a, "Poly Drug Abuse—The Response of the Medical Profession and the Pharmaceutical Industry." Report of the (House) Select Committee on Narcotics Abuse and Control, Washington, D.C.

(Wolff) 1979b, "Women's Dependency on Prescription Drugs." Hearings before the (House) Select Committee on Narcotics Abuse and Control, Washington, D.C.

Wolpert, A. 1968, "Psychopharmacology: An Overview," *Psychiatric Quarterly,* 42:444–451.

Yacknin, E. 1978, Memorandum—"Proposed Regulations on Valium and Other Benzodiazepines." Pennsylvania Legal Services Center, November.

Zackey, J. 1980, "Valium—Hazardous Overprescription in an Anxious Society," *Trial,* 24:16–18.

Zawadski, R., Glazer, G., and Lurie, E. 1978, "Psychotropic Drug Use Among Institutionalized and Noninstitutionalized Medicaid Aged in California," *Journal of Gerontology,* 33:825–834.

INDEX

ABOUT THE AUTHOR

Mickey C. Smith is Professor of Health Care Administration at the School of Pharmacy of the University of Mississippi in Oxford, where he has taught since 1966. Prior to his academic experience, he served as marketing manager for a pharmaceutical firm and practiced community pharmacy.

Dr. Smith has written and edited several textbooks in pharmacy, notably, *Principles of Pharmaceutical Marketing* and *Pharmacy, Drugs and Medical Care*, each of which has appeared in multiple editions. His research and professional writings have been published in nearly 100 different pharmacy, medical, and social science journals. He has received national awards for research and leadership in education.

Dr. Smith holds B.S. (pharmacy) and M.S. degrees from the St. Louis College of Pharmacy. His Ph.D. degree was received from the University of Mississippi.